THE NICARAGUAN REVOLUTION IN HEALTH

THE NICARAGUAN REVOLUTION IN HEALTH
From Somoza to the Sandinistas

JOHN M. DONAHUE

Bergin & Garvey Publishers, Inc.
MASSACHUSETTS

First published in 1986 by
Bergin & Garvey Publishers, Inc.
670 Amherst Road
South Hadley, Massachusetts 01075

Copyright © 1986 by Bergin & Garvey Publishers, Inc. All rights reserved. No part of this publication may be reproduced or transmitted in any form or by any means, electronic or mechanical, including photocopy, recording or any information storage or retrieval system, without permission in writing from the publisher.

6789   987654321

Library of Congress Cataloging-in-Publication Data

Donahue, John M.
    The Nicaraguan revolution in health.

    Bibliography: p.
    Includes index.
    1. Medical care—Nicaragua—History. 2. Public health—Nicaragua—History. 3. Nicaragua—Social conditions. 4. Nicaragua—History—1979-   . I. Title. [DNLM: 1. Delivery of Health Care—trends—Nicaragua. 3. Health Policy—trends—Nicaragua. WA 540 DN5 D6n]
RA454.N5D66 1986   362.1′097285   85-31562
ISBN 0-89789-101-5

Manufactured in the United States of America.

*Dedicated to the children
of
Nicaragua and the United States
especially
Arnoldo, Aldo and Alexia
and
Edward and Bernadette*

CONTENTS

	Preface	xi
	Introduction by Lambros Comitas	xv
CHAPTER 1	Health Care and Social Change	1
CHAPTER 2	Health Care Before the Revolution	9
CHAPTER 3	The Insurrection and After: The Sandinista Program	23
CHAPTER 4	Popular Education in Health	63
CHAPTER 5	Competing Agendas in Primary Health Care	87
CHAPTER 6	Conclusion: Lessons for the Future	99
APPENDIX A	Health Education Pamphlets	103
APPENDIX B	Popular Health Documents	133
	References	139
	Index	151

LIST OF TABLES

Table 3.1	Summary Statistics of the 1981 Popular Health Campaigns	32
Table 3.2	Number of Persons Vaccinated and Doses Provided in Nicaragua for the Years 1980, 1981, 1982 and 1983	33
Table 3.3	Transmittable Diseases Reported in Nicaragua and Rates per 100,000 Inhabitants 1980, 1981, 1982, 1983 and 1984	35
Table 3.4	Number of Medical Encounters in Nicaragua by Health Region and Special Zone for the Years 1977, 1980, 1981, 1982 and 1983	44
Table 3.5	Distribution of Physicians in Nicaragua by Health Region and Special Zones for the Years 1980, 1982 and 1983	47
Table 3.6	Hospital Capacity and Usage in Nicaragua 1977, 1980, 1981, 1982, 1983, 1984	49
Table 3.7	Hospital Bed Capacity in Nicaragua 1977, 1980, 1981, 1982 and 1984	50
Table 3.8	Medical Encounters in Nicaragua in Health Centers and Hospitals 1980, 1981, 1982 and 1983	53
Table 3.9	Health Clinics and Health Posts in Nicaragua by Health Regions and Special Zones for the Years 1980, 1981 and 1982	54
Table 3.10	Dental Encounters in Nicaragua 1977, 1980, 1981, 1982 and 1983	55

LIST OF FIGURES

Figure 3.1	Map of Nicaragua	28
Figure 3.2	Structure of Popular Participation in Health in Nicaragua	30
Figure 3.3	Number of Doses Provided in Nicaragua for the Years 1980, 1981, 1982 and 1983	34
Figure 3.4	Cases of Transmittable Diseases Reported in Nicaragua 1980, 1981, 1982, 1983 and 1984	36
Figure 3.5	Number of Medical Encounters in Nicaragua by Health Region and Special Zone for the Years 1977, 1980, 1981 and 1982	45
Figure 3.6	Distribution of Physicians in Nicaragua by Health Region and Special Zones for the Years 1980 and 1982	48
Figure 3.7	Changes in Hospital Bed Capacity in Nicaragua 1977 and 1982, 1982 and 1984	51

PREFACE

This book will be published almost ten years to the month after I first began a study of health delivery in Nicaragua. I had been in Latin America since 1966 when I first began work as a Maryknoll Missioner in the Institute of Rural Education on the Altiplano of Peru. Subsequent fieldwork in southern Colombia as a graduate student at Columbia University in Applied Anthropology raised more questions as to why rural peoples faced such major obstacles in their development. My first opportunity to view the development process from the point of view of national governments and international development agencies came in 1976 and again in 1978 when I was a consultant in rural health delivery to the United States Agency for International Development (USAID) Mission in Bolivia. My education in the politics of health began then, too. As a consultant to USAID, my task was to train Nicaraguan health educators in the application of social science theory and methods to rural health delivery. As I accompanied the health educators into the rural villages in northern Nicaragua and spoke with the peasants, it became acutely clear that the major obstacle to their health and well-being was the political economy of the dictatorship, as enforced by the National Guard. Many of the peasants and some of the health educators themselves were sympathizers of the Sandinista Front of National Liberation (FSLN) which was operating in the region.

Events have moved quickly in Nicaragua. When I returned after the revolution in March 1980, I met some of my former students in health education who were working in the newly created National Unified Health System. On that and subsequent visits, we traveled back to some of the villages where they had worked before the revolution. During an academic leave from Trinity University in 1982 and during the next two summers, I continued research on the changes in health policy and practice in both urban and rural areas. I found that the health sector provides a unique "window" through which to view the revolutionary process as it unfolds over time. Contrary to declarations about the dangers of totalitarianism in Nicaragua, I observed that many of the revolution's changes in health, as in other areas such as defense, education and the agrarian reform, were *negotiated*. I have attempted to document that process in the health sector, especially as it occurs at the grass-roots level through popular organization and participation.

From an anthropological perspective, the Nicaraguan revolution represents a cultural, and in some respects a religious, revitalization movement (Wallace 1956). This is not to deny the geopolitical significance of the Nicaraguan revolution for other Central American countries and for its neighbor to the north, the United States. Wallace (1956:274) notes that most revitalization movements, if they are to be successful, must come to grips with political resistance, be it domestic or international. He notes that strategies of adaptation include doctrinal modification, political and diplomatic maneuver, and force. These strategies are not mutually exclusive nor are they necessarily maintained throughout the life of the movement. Instances of each can be found in the Nicaraguan revitalization during the past five years.

Current political commentary in the United States often seeks to represent Nicaragua as a pawn of foreign powers, bent upon the expansion of their influence into the Americas. To reduce the Nicaraguan revolution to the status of pawn in a larger geopolitical chess game betrays a "zero-sum" and reductionist political world view. This view, to be logically coherent, must deny or explain away the indigenous character of cultural revitalizations in the Third World.

Another alternative would be to accept the reasons for the revitalization as justified and seek to identify with the legitimate goals of the revolution in social and economic development. This would mean that the United States would have to work with the leaders of the Sandinista revolution. Wallace (1956:274) would argue that the "charismatic leadership" characteristic of revitalization movements is as much a function of the group which recognizes the "prophet" as it is of the individual himself. The vast majority of Nicaraguan people support the reforms in health, education and the agrarian economy and support the leaders who envisioned and initiated the changes.

The eventual success of the Nicaraguan revolution will depend on how well the American people and government recognize the fundamentally popular character of that revolution and allow it the political space to internally adapt to a loyal opposition and culturally transform itself.

This book describes how this process of adaptation and transformation is underway in the health field and suggests that, given the opportunity, the same process of popular organization and participation could revitalize the whole of Nicaraguan society.

ACKNOWLEDGMENTS

This book, as a final product, is the author's sole responsibility. Yet, many people have contributed to this effort and without their assistance, criticism and even friendly debate, it could not have been completed.

Arnoldo and Rosario Toruno and their children were most hospitable and opened their home to me on several occasions. Arnoldo Toruno, Carlos Lopez and Paulino Castellon, all with the Ministry of Health, insured that I had access to a wide range of data and opinion. Graciela Pechersky, an Argentinian anthropologist and Roberto Capote, a Cuban health planner with the Pan American Health Organization, provided friendly debate on health strategies at work in Nicaragua. Richard Garfield offered helpful criticisms on some earlier drafts of this research. Tom Bossert, James Morrissey and Antonio Ugalde provided careful suggestions and recommendations on the issues of national health planning and medical professionalism. Several colleagues at Trinity University should be recognized. Ken Kramer, my former Dean, encouraged my early research in Nicaragua and Tom Greaves, the current Dean, continued that support. Acknowledgement must be made of Trinity University and the Faculty Development Committee, for funding this research in times of increasing political polarization in the United States over the issue of American foreign policy towards Nicaragua. A special word of recognition is due my editor, Michael Coffey, whose suggestions added clarity and precision to the manuscript. My wife, Simone Laudumiey, merits more than these few words, for she is herself *una compa*, as the Nicaraguans would say, who has shared the struggles of research whether I was walking the hills of Nicaragua or sitting in front of the word processor. Finally, acknowledgement must be made to those many health educators and community health workers, too numerous to name, who shared with me their experiences in trying to provide health to all the people. This is really their book.

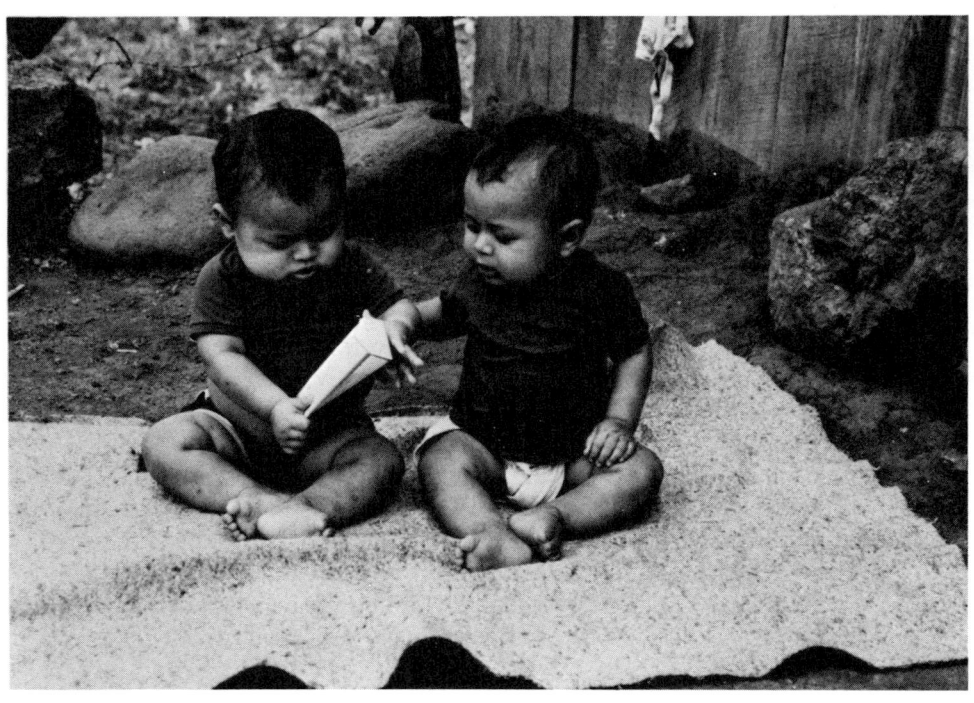
These twin boys embody the results of increased well-baby care in the rural areas of Nicaragua.

INTRODUCTION

With the fall of the Somoza regime in 1979 and the ascendency of the Sandinistas, the nature of Nicaraguan society began to be transformed. In the few years that have elapsed, shifts of systemic proportion are altering the social landscape of this turbulent and much bedeviled nation and dramatically affecting the lives of its citizens. Core institutions that function to regulate society such as the armed forces, police, and the courts have metamorphosed to meet different societal needs and exigencies; agrarian reform and cooperative ventures are changing the institutional contours of the rural economy; the massive national literacy campaign and the formation of popular education centers have expanded opportunities for education; and the health system, once essentially restricted to urban areas, has been energetically spread throughout the country. It is this latter subject, the development of the Nicaraguan health system, which is probed — in detail and free of ideological bias — in this timely book by Professor John M. Donahue. The author, a gifted anthropologist and Latin Americanist, explores the changes taken place in the health system since 1979 within the context of revolutionary change and examines the process by which that health system made to conform to a totally new political environment. In both these tasks he has succeeded admirably.

For the public health specialist, Professor Donahue offers a full and precise study of the process by which the health system of a poor Central American nation is radically reorganized, reoriented and rejuvenated over a short period of time. Pre-revolutionary Nicaragua with high morbidity and mortality was badly serviced by a neglected, fragmented health system controlled from the top. Political crises and eventual success in toppling the dictatorship set the scene for significant changes: planning and setting priorities for restructuring the health system; forging the nationwide health organizations; selecting and training the *brigadistas*; launching the massive health campaigns and developing specialized health programs; dealing with the issue of professional versus popular control of the health system and with tensions between rural and urban areas; and, finally, developing effective popular health education, a theme given considerable attention by the author.

All in all, this is a dramatic story, well-recounted in the pages that follow. More importantly, however, the value of this book is that it is not necessarily localized to Nicaragua. Although its insights and findings are obviously grounded in the Nicaraguan experience, the grave health problems and the measures selected to solve these problems are not, in essence, unique to Nicaragua but similar, in many ways, to those commonly found in Third World countries under no revolutionary pressure. Often the causes of such problems are homologous. As a study of the process used to develop a health system, the book provides lessons of undoubted and lasting value.

Readers more generally interested in contemporary Nicaragua as an ideological or geopolitical vortex in international politics should be cautioned not to set *The Nicaraguan Revolution in Health* casually aside as some specialized monograph on some basically non-controversial, scientific theme. In fact, I would strongly maintain that the very subject of this book and its manner of presentation provide the careful reader with a particularly useful vantage point from which to begin to unravel the internal complexities of revolutionary Nicaragua. The Sandinista health system, molded as it has been by ideology and competing pressures from the center, the regions, and the localities, and buffeted almost continuously from the outside by counter-revolutionary activity is, from my theoretical perspective, a veritable microcosm, a reflection of the larger, still forming revolutionary society that encompasses it. Consequently, to comprehend the process of development and present state of the Nicaraguan health system is to open a window on the emerging structure of that nation. Linked to this, but from Professor Donahue's developmental perspective, the transformation of the Nicaraguan health system is well underway and, given the opportunity, the same process of popular organization and participation that spurred developments in the health field "could revitalize the whole of Nicaraguan society."

I met John Donahue in the late 1960s in La Paz, Bolivia, when he was a Maryknoll Missioner on assignment as community action advisor to a very large number of Aymara Indian communities in Juli on the Peruvian side of Lake Titicaca. As I remember our first meetings, we discussed the various graduate departments of political science to which he could apply. Although I should like to think that my advice on that subject was objective and straightforward, I am also aware that subliminally, if not otherwise, I trumpeted the virtues of my own discipline, anthropology. Whether or not these messages influenced John Donahue, I will, nonetheless, very happily take credit for his decision to study anthropology. In 1970, he entered the Joint Program in Applied Anthropology at Teachers College, Columbia University. He received the Doctor of Philosophy degree in 1975 after successfully defending his excellent dissertation on circular and return aspects of labor migration in southern Colombia. Over his professional years, he has earned the reputation as a superior field researcher and an anthropologist of note for his substantial work in Peru, Colombia, Bolivia, and Nicaragua. A member of the faculty of Trinity University, San Antonio, Texas, for a decade and now Professor of Anthropology at that institution, Professor Donahue deserves commendation for *The Nicaraguan Revolution in Health* not only for its contributions to the understanding of change in systems but for its practical value to the people and governments of Nicaragua and the Third World.

LAMBROS COMITAS
Teachers College, Columbia University

THE NICARAGUAN REVOLUTION IN HEALTH

Chapter 1
HEALTH CARE AND SOCIAL CHANGE

Health systems research inevitably leads to an analysis of the larger sociopolitical structure of which health delivery is a reflection (Mott 1974). The link between political structure and health delivery is the topic of an increasing number of studies (Anderson, Smedly, and Anderson 1970; Baer 1982; Danielson 1975,1979; Elling 1980; Elling and Kerr 1975; Navarro 1976,1977,1980; New and New 1975; Roemer 1969,1976; Ronaghy and Solten 1974; Starr 1982; UNICEF/WHO 1977).

The Executive Board of the World Health Organization, in a statement made over ten years ago, called attention to the fact that few or no examples exist "where a change in emphasis of the type and degree required has been introduced within an exisiting health service without a preceding change in social policies." "This link between health service and political structure," they continue, "is not so intimate that the health services cannot change separately and independently within most sociopolitical systems. However, the manner in which health services change in different systems and under different circumstances, <u>the process of change</u>, and the dominating constraints making change difficult are largely unknown" (WHO 1973:110, italics mine).

Changes in the Nicaraguan Health System since the Revolution of July 1979 provide an excellent case study of the process through which a health system is made to conform to a new political environment. The purpose of this book is to describe and interpret these changes within the context of revolutionary change. Revolutions are dynamic and often unchartered, so special attention is given to the course of events which suggest how changes in the health system were negotiated.

METHODS OF ANALYSIS

To study the process of change in a health system, Firth's distinction between structure and organization is useful (Firth 1963:35-36). Structure implies ordered and predictable sets of social relationships that are related as parts to a whole. An example of a structural analysis in the comparative study of national health systems is Roemer (1977:21-22). He identifies five principal types of health systems ranging from free enterprise to socialist models. Typological approaches to the cross-national study of health systems rely on a structural-functional model of analysis. They are useful for identifying the points of change in health systems. A "before and after" structural analysis may indicate that change has taken place, but it does not address the process whereby the change took place.

Firth argues that a structural analysis alone cannot interpret social change. He concludes that "analysis of the organizational aspect of social action is the necessary complement to analysis of the structural aspect" (1963:36). Social structure and social organization are reciprocal elements in the study of social change. A health system as a social structure can be described as a set of group relations or of ideal types. As a social organization, a health system comprises the concrete activities of individuals and groups as they pursue specific goals. A processual methodology focuses upon the choices of actors within a structure or among various structures in a given field of activity. As a field of activity, a health system might contain several alternative goals among which actors might compete as they seek to effect the internal configuration of the system. In a revolutionary society the actors might have a wider range of choices because the old structures are being redefined.

Elling (1980:102-105) describes the links between political structure and health systems in terms of health planning. He identifies three characteristics of health planning that would indicate change towards an ideal health system: a comprehensive health plan, coordination with national goals other than health, and broad popular participation. Since decision-making depends upon the organization of authority, Elling categorizes authority structures by the degree of concentration of power (centralized vs. decentralized) and the degree of solidarity of political action (concerted vs. fractional). He argues that a concerted-decentralized structure is "likely to be most supportive of the regionalized and otherwise ideal health and medical care system" (1980:107). He says that a health system and the political economy in which it is embedded change in accordance with internal pressures and their place in the world system (1980:107).

THE CASE OF NICARAGUA

Nicaragua offers a unique setting in which to analyze the effect of changes in the political economy on the health delivery system. When the National Government of Reconstruction created the National Unified Health System (SNUS) three weeks after the revolution of July 19, 1979, the objective was clear. The health system was to be an integral part of the effort to create a participatory democracy within a socialist political economy (MINSA 1982a:1-12,53-57).

The newly created national health system in Nicaragua represents a definite structural change. Yet, to quickly label a health system within a revolutionary society "socialist" may be precipitous. Segall (1983:221-225) recommends an approach in which observable institutional arrangements and behaviors are employed to determine the fit between political structures and health care systems. One should focus upon the outcomes of decision-making, class and status group struggles, and institutional realignments within the health system and within the larger political economy. This approach, similar to that which Firth recommends, would entail an analysis of the institutional actors, competing goals, and negotiated outcomes. If indeed a health system is moving in the direction of a socialist structure, Segall notes several empirical indicators of that movement: 1) emphasis on the social etiology of disease and efforts to enhance health through a more equal access to goods and services; 2) programatic efforts to encourage participation in and organization of health-related activities; and 3) empowerment of the people to take economic and political control of health services out of the exclusive domain of professionals.

In this last regard, Navarro (1977), in his study of the Soviet health system, concludes that a nationalized rather than a socialized health system has emerged in that country's health sector. A nationalized health system is controlled ultimately by a managerial bureaucracy that denies direct input from the community. He understands the one can be a step to the other if the nationalized system ultimately leads to popular involvement, participation, and control over the health institution.

The nature of professional dominance in health (Freidson 1970, 1984) suggests that the transition from a nationalized to a socialized system would not be without conflict. In the developing world where health needs are primarily preventive, the conflict is for professional or popular control over the organization and delivery of health services, especially for primary health care in rural areas. The outcome of that conflict is what eventually shapes the internal configuration of any health system in the developing world. I argue that the issue of professional dominance does not disappear as a health system changes from a private to a nationalized or even to a socialized system (Lampton 1974, New 1984). The reason for this lies in the way that the medical profession is organized.

Freidson (1970:154) argues that professional dominance arises from the structure of the occupation itself. Medical professionals must pursue their careers in "concrete, historically located institutions" (1970:155). In addition, professionals' pride in their work often translates into an attitude of superiority over other health occupations and lay clients. As a result, he concludes that "since those weaknesses stem from professionalism itself, professions cannot be expected to be able to rectify them"(1970:156).

One might ask how medical professionalism can be reconciled with popular participation in health care delivery. Marie R. Haug (1973, 1975, 1977) argues that professions in the United States are losing their prestige and authority as consumers become more knowledgeable and better organized in the health care field. Freidson (1984) disagrees with the "deprofessionalization thesis." He argues that "community and self-help groups have a high mortality rate and often a highly transient group of participants" (1984:7). He notes the importance of the consumer movement of the 1970s, but is not convinced that over time "the professions are losing their relative prestige and respect, their expertise or their monopoly over the exercise of that expertise" (1984:8). The medical profession in Nicaragua is undergoing change as a result of the nationalization of health services in 1979 and increased citizen participation in health planning and delivery of services. The controversy over professional dominance in Nicaragua might shed light on similar processes in other developing countries and in the United States itself. Indeed, an analysis of this conflict provides insight into how a health system becomes socialist in name and reality.

Changes in the larger political economy since 1979 reveal that Nicaragua is moving in the direction of a socialist structure. National reforms in defense, education, the agrarian economy and health have provided Nicaraguans with increased access to goods and services. New social groups have emerged as a result of the reforms. Somoza's professional army was completely replaced by the Sandinista army and police. New peasant organizations emerged out of the agrarian reform. On-going literacy programs rely heavily upon volunteer instructors in the rural villages. By contrast, a major professional class carried over into the health sector of the revolutionary society. Many physicians had actively participated in the insurrection and supported the Sandinistas in the overthrow of Somoza. After the revolution, the professional interests of physicians in the curative and institutional dimensions of the new national health system did not reflect the epidemiological reality of the country. They sought modes of community participation which enhance utilization of services but do not challenge their control over planning and delivery functions. Accordingly, within primary care medical professionals tend to emphasize institutional care more than outreach, and professional control over paraprofessionals and nonprofessionals. By and large, medical professionals within the Ministry represent interests that are best accommodated within a nationalized and not a socialized health system.

The Sandinista revolution places high priority on community participation in the national reforms. The history of primary health care efforts in Nicaragua illustrate that community participation served very different purposes within the political economy of the Somoza dictatorship and that of the Sandinista government (see Chapter 2). The public health campaigns in Nicaragua subsequent to the revolution of 1979 relied heavily on mass

6   The Nicaraguan Revolution in Health

popular organization and participation. The success of the efforts motivated the World Health Organization and UNICEF to choose that country as a model primary health care system (see Chapter 3). There continues a struggle within the Ministry of Health between advocates of a populist approach to participation and those who prefer more institutionalist strategies. At the normative level, citizen participation is not necessarily a threat to professional or bureaucratic dominance. The conflicts and challenges may often take place not at the level of goals, but at the level of means (Freidson 1970:130-131).

Scholars point out that definitions of community participation are open to different ideological interpretations and include a wide range of implementing strategies. In the field of cooperative organizations Korten has observed that development programs fail because "they are often creations of the government to provide government control over production and marketing rather than voluntary creations of individuals to increase collective market power" (1982:4). Likewise, community participation in health programs often functions as a form of social control and legitimization of a political regime (Keyzer and Ulate 1980, Ugalde 1981). When organized communities in Panama began to make demands upon the government for increased health care, the government abandoned the health program (Ugalde 1981:17). Community participation, then, is no guarantee that governments will respond with the political will and allocation of resources necessary to meet the goal. Moreover, the concept of community participation is so broad that it is compatible with quite divergent political economies for a variety of different functions, ranging from national and regional health planning to local financing and delivery of services to simply generating greater utilization of existing clinical services.

Advocates of community control in Nicaragua emphasize participation in and control of local health delivery and stress health promotion through popular strategies and outreach rather than an institutionally based delivery of services. Conversely nonprofessional and volunteer community health workers and health educators seek participation strategies that emphasize primary health care delivery in noninstitutionalized settings and health programs at the community level. They argue for grass roots participation in health planning and delivery. This includes both the mass dissemination of health knowledge, especially in the area of disease prevention and the involvement of volunteer workers from the community trained in simplified medicine (see

Chapter 4). Health educators, paraprofessionals, and community health workers represent interests that are better served in a socialized health system.

Backers of each approach seek to influence decision-making in the Ministry of Health in favor of their particular model of community health care and participation strategies. The discussion in Chapter 5 focuses on the conflict within the SNUS between those who seek professional control over health delivery and community participation and those who argue for a more community controlled health care system.

The Nicaraguan Revolution in health and in its other dimensions as well, is best understood as a process of negotiation and becoming. This book will describe how the Nicaraguan Revolution and subsequent changes in the political economy allowed professional and popular constituencies to compete within the health system. The significance of the conflict lies in the fact that even in a health system characterized by a high degree of political will, there continues a struggle between advocates of professional and popular agendas. The most important feature of the Nicaraguan health system may be the process itself, if that proves to turn professionals from domination to cooperation with the organized people.

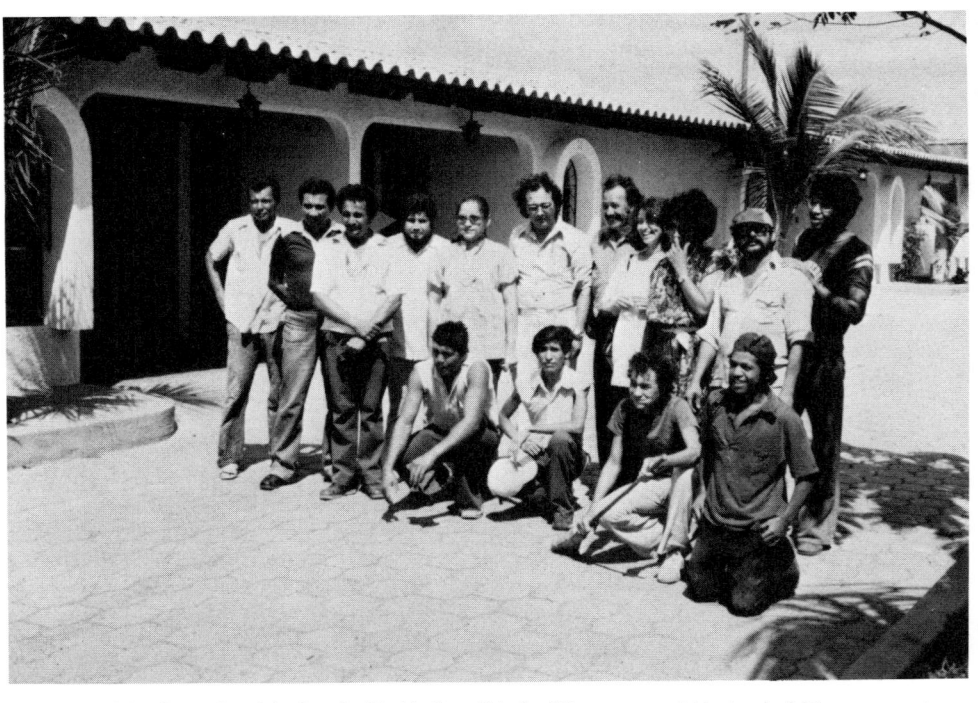

One of the first tasks of the Popular Health Council in La Primavera, a neighborhood of Managua, was to convert a former brothel into a maternity clinic.

Chapter 2
HEALTH CARE BEFORE THE REVOLUTION

An analysis of health conditions and reform measures before the revolution serves two purposes. (1) First, we can observe the links between health care and the political economy of the dictatorship. Second, a discussion of prerevolutionary community health programs will set the stage for an evaluation of the changes introduced into the health system after July 1979.

HEALTH CONDITIONS

Between 1942 and 1959 various sectors of the Nicaraguan work force became organized as a result of the expansion of commercial agriculture, industry, and the state bureacracy. The Social Security System was introduced to provide health services for these workers. By 1978 the Nicaraguan Social Security Institute (INSS) served 8.4 percent of the total population and 16 percent of the economically active population (MINSA 1981b:13). Among these, the INSS provided services to the service sector, mainly government workers (66 percent), industrial workers (28 percent) and to a small percentage of agricultural workers (2.7 percent). In 1974 the INSS captured 39 percent of the Nicaraguan Health Sector Budget and actually spent 50.4 percent (USAID 1976:46). The Ministry of Health had primary responsibility for the entire population of Nicaragua and sole responsibility for the rural population. In 1974 the Ministry of Health (MOH) budget accounted for only 16 percent of health sector expenditures (excluding the water and sewer agency) (USAID 1976:46). Of this 81 percent went to operating expenses. Nearly 75 percent of the budget was spent in Managua which accounted for only 25 percent of the entire population in 1972 (USAID 1976:81). The effect of these allocation policies was to leave the vast majority of Nicaraguans, especially those in rural areas, to make do with what meager resources were available in the private or traditional health sectors. As might be expected, the result of such a misallocation of health resources was reflected in morbidity and mortality rates.

Studies by the Institute of Nutrition for Central America and Panama (INCAP) in 1969 and 1975 found that 57 percent of children less than 5 years of age suffered from some degree of malnutrition (USAID 1976: 105, 185). In fact, between 1965 and 1975 the percentage of children in the second and third degrees of malnutrition increased 105.2 percent, from 50 to 102 per 1000 (Teller 1981:11). Yet malnutrition was clearly class specific. The INCAP nutritional survey in 1966 revealed that "per capita consumption for the lower 50% of the population averages 1767 calories and 46.6 grams of protein per day while the upper class consumes an average of 3931 calories and 111.9 grams of protein per capita per day" (USAID 1976:193). Hospital data from 1970 reveals that the maternal mortality rate stood at 137 per 100,000 live births. Estimates for the rural areas reached 280 per 100,000 live births (USAID 1976:105). In 1975, 60,000 or more births, plus 70 percent of all child care, were estimated to have taken place outside the Nicaraguan health system. In rural areas almost 80 percent of manpower needs were met by <u>parteras</u> and <u>curanderos</u> (2) with no public sector support (USAID 1976:116). As a result of poor nutrition and lack of maternal-child care programs, infant mortality rates reached 149 per 1000 live births in 1979 (PAHO 1979). Deaths of children age 4 and under accounted for 32.3 percent of all deaths in 1975 (USAID 1976:104).

Morbidity patterns reflect the causes of such high infant mortality. Under-reporting makes it difficult to gauge with accuracy the actual occurrence of communicable diseases. For example, in 1974 only 852 cases of measles, and only 104 deaths, were reported (Division of Biostatistics, Nicaragua Ministry of Health, 1975; reported in USAID 1976:132). Yet the authors of the Health Sector

Assessment note that vitually all children in Central America give evidence of a previous infection of measles by the age of 10 (USAID 1976:133). The true incidence of measles would then approach the birth rate minus children who die before being exposed to the disease. They conclude that in Nicaragua, with approxmimately 84,000 live births a year and about 9,000 infant deaths per year, there should be nearly 75,000 cases of measles reported per year (USAID 1976:133).

Morbidity patterns among adults included endemic goiter, which affected between 30 and 39 percent of the entire population (PAHO 1979). In 1976, 45,400 cases of parasitosis were reported along with 22,400 cases of diarrhea. This made enteritis the major cause of general and infant mortality in the country (MINSA 1980a:17; USAID 1976:168). In 1978, potable water services reached only 41.4 percent of the urban population and 10.9 percent of rural people. In the same year only 29.4 percent of the urban population was connected to sanitary sewage disposal systems or to septic tanks. In the rural areas some 828,000 people did not even have latrines (MINSA 1980a:17;USAID 1976:168). Yet, in 1968 the amount allocated for water and sewage projects amounted to only 5.6 percent of the total Public Health budget (Navarro, n.d.).

Two other diseases from which the youth were particularly at risk were tetanus and poliomyelitis. From 1951 to 1979 Nicaragua experienced polio outbreaks every two to three years. In 1974 a total of 200,697 doses of polio vaccine were administered to children 4 years old and under. This represented 17 percent of the population at risk (USAID 1976:131). While polio was not a major cause of death, it did leave a whole cohort of handicapped persons who continued to need medical attention. On the other hand, tetanus ranked as a leading cause of death among children and left many susceptible to a host of other illnesses. In 1974 three innoculations, for diptheria, pertussis, and tetanus (DPT), covered only 5.7 percent of the population at risk under 4 years of age (USAID 1976:134).

The overall failure of the Ministry of Health to address the severe public health problems of the majority population is rooted in the prerevolutionary health system. The system was characterized by vertical control, fragmentation within the 23 autonomous institutions making up the health sector, and a mode of community organization which enhanced the control and fragmentation.

HEALTH PROGRAMS UNDER SOMOZA

The concentration of political power by the Somoza family over a 45-year period is well documented (Millett 1977; Booth 1985). The extension of the Somoza family's verticial control over the agricultural, industrial, and banking institutions was notorious. By the mid 1970s the Somoza family contolled 21 percent of all agricultural land (CIERA 1982:9). The Somoza Banking Group extracted funds from the state and its autonomous institutions, such as the National Bank and the Social Security System, to finance capital investments in construction materials, meat packing, tobacco products, shoes, rice production, real estate, mass media, auto parts, and auto sales (Booth 1985:81). After the earthquake of 1972 Somoza became infamous for the expropriation of international relief assistance for personal gain. His personal fortune in 1974 was estimated to be nearly $400 million (Booth 1985:81). Somoza's ability to garner such wealth was based upon a system of vertical control. The control was exercised through political patronage in which benefits within the system were allocated to enhance dependency on the dictator. (3) The National Guard was itself the major beneficiary and enforcer of the patronage system.

The patronage system had direct effects on the health sector. Before the revolution only about 28 percent of the population had regular access to health care. Of the health resources made available by Somoza 90 percent went to 10 percent of the population (Halperin and Garfield 1982:388). The authors of the Health Sector Assessment sum up the major effect of the Somoza dictatorship on the health sector.

> The long history of one party rule in the country... resulted in a centralized decision making process with limited delegation of responsibility and authority which often required the President to personally intervene in issues affecting even small amounts of sector resources. Thus the health sector and many health sector personnel lacked the motivation and innovative-experimental approach necessary to make a major impact on the enormous health problems facing the health agencies with limited resources.... Additionally when considering health policy in Nicaragua one must always keep closely attuned to the pronouncements and speeches of the

President. A strong executive tradition with little legislative or health agency independence of action previously meant that health policy decisions at most levels needed executive approval prior to change or implementation. This pattern of executive decision making in health was re-enforced by the lack of planning and management skills present in the health sector [USAID 1976:6,13-14].

One could argue that the fragmentation of the health sector itself was a dimension of vertical political control. The presence of many competing health institutions diffused internal solidarity within the health sector and left each entity dependent on political patronage and control from above. As will be subsequently shown, Somoza allocated health benefits less on the criteria of need and more on the basis of strategic and political impact. The multiplicity of health institutions allowed Somoza greater flexibility in granting rewards to those groups who demonstrated support or in attempts to quiet dissent. In two instances community health programs were placed in rural areas where the peasants were sympathetic to the guerrilla opposition. (4)

The 23 separate institutions that comprised the public health sector included the Ministry of Public Health (MSP), the National Social Assistance and Welfare Board (JNAPS), which had responsibility for "national hospitals," and some 19 local Social Welfare Boards (JLAS), which operated departmental hospitals, the Social Security Institute (INSS), and the Military Hospital. (5)

Each of the 23 organizations remained nearly autonomous in the areas of financing and budgetary control. As a consequence, the major National Health Plans lacked a clear mandate and integrated approach. The First National Health Plan covered the years 1965-1974. An evaluation of the Plan in 1971 "found little implementation due to scarce financial resources, lack of trained personnel and insufficient administrative support" (USAID 1976:9). The Second National Health Plan 1976-1980, formulated in 1975, was abbreviated by the Revolution. It did not include the National Hospital Systems (JNAPS) and the Social Security Institute (INSS). The Plan was only directed to the Ministry of Health whose budget barely represented 16 percent of the health sector expenditures (USAID 1976:46). Vertical control and ineffective planning were reflected in several evaluations made of health delivery services during the 1970s. An internal study of the National Hospital System's 25 facilities in 1973 found "a combination of poor physical plant, lack of equipment, uncleanliness and poor quality of medical attention.... Fifteen hospitals lacked proper hygiene, adequate preventive medicine programs and effective plant and equipment maintenance. Nineteen hospitals lacked any emergency facilities, a basic means of access of local patients to hospital services" (USAID 1976:10). The lack of emergency rooms in three of four hospitals effectively excluded the local populace from primary care and out-patient ambulatory services.

The system of vertical control benefited from institutional fragmentation and made for ineffective hospital health delivery. It also left its mark on community participation in other areas of the public health sector.

In 1973 Practical Concepts, Inc., an independent health systems contractor, conducted an evaluation of the 55 health centers built during 1968 and 1973 with an AID loan. "The major conclusion seemed to be that no provisions were made to provide these centers, once built, with adequate personnel, supplies and management support" (USAID 1976:9). Utilization rates were low and yet only 9.4 percent of services were given outside the centers. Outreach and community participation were at a minimum. The authors of the Health Sector Assessment conclude that

> generally the center is seen by the community as an extension of the MOH in Managua and that the MOH maintains control from the national level... With the exception of the large health centers in urban areas, there are few community boards that direct a health center... It is unfortunate that such Boards do not play a greater role because of their potential in generating community support and in managing the health center's operations (USAID 1976:94).

In fact, the lack of broad-based community participation in the health sector resulted in little accountability of the health professionals to the community. A 1974 Ministry of Health personnel manpower efficiency study quoted in the Health Sector Assessment indicated "that the average health center was operating at about 40 percent capacity in terms of patient visits per medical hour (standard of 6 patients per hour)" (USAID 1976:109).

THE ROLE OF USAID

Mention was made earlier of the USAID loan of $2.2 million dollars in 1965 to set up 55 health centers. The loan document, Health Centers-Rural Mobile Health, 524-L-023, also provided for the continuation and strengthening of the Rural Mobile Health Program (PUMAR) designed to provide outreach into rural areas, and the incorporation of newly graduated physicians and other medical personnel into the program under the obligatory Social Service Law of Nicaragua (USAID 1976:252).

By 1973 the underutilization and inefficiency of the program prompted USAID to propose grants which would seek to address the two problem areas. Rural Community Health Services Grant 524-15-530-110 would seek to increase utilization by organizing community participation. Rural Health Institutional Development Grant 524-11-530-114 would focus on management training to enhance planning and more efficient administration of rural health programs (USAID 1976:253-257). The Rural Community Health Program (PRACS-Programa Rural de Accion Communitaria en Salud) approved in December 1975 had as its purpose:

To stimulate participation of the population in the development and implementation of health programs through the formation of village health committees to oversee the delivery of health information, health services, and simplified medicine to the rural, isolated population through the development of an effective and efficient cadre of community level health workers and through the integration of health related governmental and voluntary agency activities at the community level (USAID 1976:254)

In 1977 a complementary program was initiated with USAID funding. PLANSAR (Plan Nacional de Saneamiento) sought "to improve the health conditions of small rural villages (50 to 300 inhabitants) through the installation of water wells equipped with hand pumps, construction of small aqueducts and latrines as well as develop vaccination programs in the communities" (Ministry of Health-PLANSAR 1977, quoted in MINSA 1981a:21, author's translation). In addition, the PLANSAR program envisioned the improvement and extension of health personnel in the rural area and the development of a patient referral system of medical facilities for social welfare.

The programs of PUMAR, PRACS, and PLANSAR represent the major antecedents of the Reform Movement of 1976 and were to serve as models for extension of the Public Health Reform throughout the country in the succeeding years.

Reliance on health facilities rather than health programs further alienated the public health institutions from the community. "Maternal and child care services tend to reach their level of effectiveness more as a result of institutional emphasis (hours of clinic, personnel or service time) than as a result of some finely tuned centralized program which focuses upon specific maternal and child health problems" (USAID 1976:114). As a consequence, public vaccination programs, for the most part, were reactive responses to outbreaks of epidemics. For example, polio vaccinations in nonepidemic years were restricted to health centers and mobile teams in rural areas. Lack of community education and involvement seriously affected distribution of the oral trivalent vaccine. In 1974 only 17 percent of children 4 years old and under were vaccinated (USAID 1976:131). The Ministry of Health did move beyond the Health Centers in the polio vaccinations of 1967, 1968, and 1971. Mass vaccinations were carried out in cantones electorales, local political offices. In 1976 this strategy was still in effect (USAID 1976:131). The result was to tie health care delivery at the local level to the vertical power structure of control and patronage.

THE REFORM MOVEMENT OF 1976

In January 1976 a seminar of high ranking Nicaraguan and American Health officials was held in Chinandega. The purpose of the meeting was "to focus attention on the need for Nicaraguan policy-makers to review and solidify health sector priorities and strategies" (USAID 1976:12). The meeting was also to allow USAID to set forth its priorities to the Nicaraguan government and seek "agreement on common grounds of interest" (USAID 1976:12). The Minister of Health summed up the strategies of the health sector and set as the first priority the control of communicable diseases in rural areas through community health projects and education. This program would include the utilization of paramedical personnel, such as parteras, (6) decentralization of health planning and administration and integration of curative and preventive health services (USAID 1976:14-15).

The concept of community organization agreed upon in the Chinandega Seminar of 1976 and concretized in the three rural health programs had several special characteristics. The major feature of the health program was its verticality. At the base of the pyramid was the Rural Health Collaborator (CRS) who "accepts voluntarily to train himself or herself and in a spirit of solidarity assumes responsibilities for the care of the individual and collective health of the community in which he/she resides" (PRACS 1977:11, my translation). The role of the CRS was to detect health problems and refer patients to health services. The CRS was also to encourage the communities to organize themselves and offer solutions which with their own resources would promote health and prevent unhealthy conditions (PRACS 1977:1). The CRS would also provide some basic health services and act "as a permanent link between health services and the communities and a doorway for the population to the health system" (PRACS 1977:1).

Placed above the CRS and acting in a supervisory capacity were the Health Educators—school teachers selected for an intensive course leading to certification in Health Education. The Health Educator was to contribute to the "active, conscious and organized participation of the community ... in which there would take place an interaction [between] educator-community and where it would be expected that the community members would consider themselves subjects and not only objects of education" (Ministry of Health, 1975, quoted in MINSA 1980a:6, my translation). In the same document, however, the vertical-broker role of the Health Educators is described. They are "to guide the population to the proposed programs inasmuch as in each program they [the Health Educator] must determine the specific actions desired of the population so that, based on those actions, the magnitude of the change produced and the methodological norms of the work of health education may be specified" (PRACS 1977, author's translation).

The verticality of the health education program tended in practice to reinforce an individualistic response to health and illness. The local, regional, national, and international structural roots of health and illness were not the focus of attention and action. Rather, attention was focused upon the lack of proper health concepts and health behavior as the basic causes of illness (Keyzer and Ulate 1980). The CRS and the Health Educator were to be salesmen of health ideas and promoters of short term communal projects. Such vertical education led the community into a false consciousness in which the causes of illness were limited to personal ignorance to be corrected by instruction in appropriate health concepts and behaviors.

The Chinandega reform sought "agreement on common grounds of interest" between USAID and Nicaraguan Health Officials. Both agreed that the major objective was "promulgation of a new organic law for the health sector, establishing a single institution combining the functions of the major existing public health agents" (USAID 1976:239). This integration did not take place under Somoza; it was finally realized in the creation of the Unified National Health System (SNUS) on August 8, 1979, three weeks after the revolution.

The failure of reform under Somoza can be traced to the dictators's use of the health system to further his political objectives. The USAID programs themselves were a part of Somoza's overall political strategy. Somoza protrayed himself to the United States as the only alternative to a communist takeover of Nicaragua. At the same time, he used American aid to advance his personal economic and political goals. When USAID-sponsored reforms suited those goals, Somoza accepted them, but always on his terms. A clear example of this is found in the USAID-funded rural health programs.

The Health Sector Assessment suggests that USAID and the MSP were at odds over the priority areas for the PRACS and PLANSAR Programs. The Agency lobbied that preference be given to Regions II (Managua) and V (Matagalpa) in part because these regions were the site of a National Agricultural Program (INVIERNO) funded by USAID. The Nicaraguan Health Sector Analysis Unit offered a recommendation that Regions IV (Nueva Segovia-Madriz) and V (Matagalpa) be the priority areas for the community development programs in health. These two areas were the scene of major guerrilla activity. The Agency concluded that "the merits of these two, and other alternative regions must be carefully weighted [sic] by the Mission, since what may be convenient politically for the Nicaraguan Government, may not necessarily fit with AID's strategy, indeed mandate, to serve the poor majority most efficiently and effectively as possible" (USAID 1976:244).

THE COMMUNITY OF CHOROTEGA

The community of Chorotega (7) is located in a mountainous zone in northwestern Nicaragua. The community has 145 homes dispersed over an area of three square kilometers. The residents live primarily from day labor on nearby farms, since little can be grown on the rocky hillsides. Some families harvest sisal from which they make hammocks for sale. The sisal is harvested twice a year. The families also buy sisal in local markets. Before the revolution of 1979 the major political figure was Don Jairo Artiaga. As <u>Juez</u> <u>de</u> <u>Mesta</u> (a local government official, appointed by Somoza), Don Jairo enjoyed much prestige. He was also the leading merchant in the community whose store was the only outlet for food stuffs brought to the community from the local town. Don Jairo's brother is an Evangelical pastor who visits the community regularly. Together they supervised the building of a small chapel for Sunday worship next to Don Jairo's house. The majority of the people of Chorotega are Catholic, but American Protestant missionaries began visiting the community several years ago. The local school teacher, Ramon Flores, is a member of that religion. He lives in the nearby town and commutes daily to the community. The American missionaires initiated the free distribution of medicines in the community. Ramon himself has some paramedical training and his wife is a nurse. By 1977 both PRACS and PLANSAR were operating in the community. A Health Committee was formed whose president was Don Jairo. Health and Education activities were subsumed under local political leadership with predictable results. On one occasion, Don Jairo, President of the Health Committee, complained that only a few members of the Committee supported the construction of a PLANSAR aqueduct from the water source on a high ridge facing his farm. Later Don Jairo pointed out that animals were drinking at a point near the source and so contaminated the water. He proposed that the community make a water trough so the animals could drink without going to the source. The suggestion received little support in the community since Don Jairo used the aqueduct to irrigate his fields. In fact, the school teacher encouraged the community to dedicate their efforts to other activities such as those benefiting the school or the distribution of medicines in the community. The CRS selected to receive training in the PRACS program was a mother in her 20s and well respected by all factions in the community. (8)

Several conclusions can be drawn from the experience of PRACS in Chorotega and the other pilot communities. The vertical mode of community participation effectively controlled the distribution of health resources through political channels. Such a pattern of distribution did little to overcome local factionalism and indeed may even have acerbated socioeconomic, political and religious divisions in the community. Health delivery and education did not engage the community directly but only as mediated by the Health Committee or the services of the CRS.

Second, the community exercised little power and was not able to hold Health Committees or officials accountable for how resources were distributed and used. Passive resistance was often the rule as evidenced in the aqueduct issue in Chorotega.

Third, whatever the reformist intentions of USAID, the Somoza Government was intent on solidifying its economic and political power at any cost. This included the violent repression of any political dissent in the very areas in which the PRACS and PLANSAR programs were operating. Given that environment, it is not surprising that in its first semester of operation PRACS was able to muster only the 16 CRS and 57 Health Committee members for a Peasant Congress (MINSA 1981a:29).

CONCLUSION

The main features of the public health system under the Somoza Government were top-down control, fragmentation, and generalized neglect. The Reform Movement of 1976 began to address the results of years of neglect, but itself was compromised by the politics of vertical control under the dictatorship. To say this and no more, however, is to miss the dynamic of change that was underway in rural Nicaraguan communities in the 1970s. We have noted the donor-recipient debate, which arose over the priority areas for the PRACS and PLANSAR programs. The Somoza Government fully realized that sympathy for the guerilla movement was strong among peasant communities in the Departments of Esteli, Matagalpa, Madriz, and Nueva Segovia. If the Government's motivation was to use health programs to offset Sandinista influence, many of the communities, CRS, and Health Educators were already Sandinista sympathizers.

The purpose of this chapter has been to place the health services and strategy of community participation within the broader context of the political economy of the Somoza dictatorship. The stage has also been set to discuss the changes, structural and organizational, which the Sandinista revolution of 1979 would initiate within the health system. The historical context will allow us to identify both the continuities and the changes in the health system as Nicaraguans rejected the dictaorship and commenced the construction of a new political economy.

NOTES

1. The health status of the Nicaraguan people prior to the Revolution of 1979 has been discussed from several points of view: Bossert 1982, 1985; Escudero 1980; Garfield and Halperin 1983; Garfield and Taboada 1984; Halperin and Garfield 1982; Holland, Davis & Gangloff 1973; INCAP 1966; Junta de Gobierno de Reconstruccion Nacional n.d.; Ministry of Health, Managua 1980b, 1981, n.d.;USAID 1976.

2. Midwives ("parteras") and healers ("curanderos") practiced among a large segment of the population but had little contact with the public health sector.

3. Vertical power relationships as mediated by "brokers" are discussed by Eric Wolf (1956) and Richard Adams (1970). Both articles can be found in Heath and Adams (1974). Dependency theory as applied to the areas of health and illness is discussed by Greaves (1982). Verticality refers here to a social relationship between two individuals or groups of unequal wealth or power in which the donor controls both the quality and quantity of the downward allocation of resources. For an extended discussion of patron-client relationships in developing countries, see Gamer (1982).

4. The Sandinista Front of National Liberation (Frente Sandinista de Liberacion Nacional-FSLN) was founded in 1961. Its 18-year history and the events which lead to its successful overthrow of the Somoza dynasty is discussed in Booth (1985:137-155). In 1976 Somoza located community health programs in the Departments of Esteli and Matagalpa which comprised the "Northern Front" of the FSLN, commanded by its founder Carlos Fonseca.

5. Within the private sector the majority of physicians (65 percent in 1974) worked full or part-time in the public institutions (MINSA 1981b:11).

6. For an analysis of this Program see Heiby (1981).

7. Place names and names of individuals have been changed to maintain anonymity.

8. The selection process in the other PRACS communities yielded mixed results. Data on the CRS selection process was available for 13 of the 16 pilot programs. Six CRS had been chosen from among several candidates, one CRS was a sole candidate and six others were chosen by default when other candidates withdrew or were disqualified. A major reason for the withdrawal of many candidates was the extended period of training (two months) away from the community.

Chapter 3
THE INSURRECTON AND AFTER: THE SANDINISTA PROGRAM

Several studies document the long and arduous history of Nicaragua under the Somoza dictatorship which began when the United States Marines ended their 22-year occupation of Nicaragua in 1933 (Walker 1982, Booth 1985). Some observers point to the earthquake of 1972 as a turning point in the fortunes of the Somoza dynasty. That earthquake virtually leveled the capital city of Managua and some 10,000 persons were killed. Millions of dollars in relief supplies, cash donations, and loans came from many countries, chiefly the United States. Yet, during the next several years the graft committed by Somoza and the National Guard in the relief effort became notorious (Millett 1977). By 1979 Somoza's economic exploitation of the country, and the repression of dissent by the National Guard during a three year "state of siege" created opposition to the dictatorship in virtually every class and social category. Before he left, Somoza plundered the National Treasury leaving only $3.5 million dollars and a foreign debt of $1.6 billion.

The insurrection (1978-1979) adversly effected even further the health of the Nicaraguan people. Over 40,000 lives were lost in a street-by-street and house-by-house struggle against the National Guard. Some 100,000 people were injured. As they retreated from a city or town, the National Guard damaged or destroyed sewage plants, water pumping and treatment plants, hospitals, and clinics. The United Nations estimated that during the war Nicaragua lost

$700 million in capital flight, $200 million in cotton exports, and $500 million dollars in physical damage, including $5 million in damages to hospitals and clinics (ECLA 1979).

Most of the damage was on the Western, or Pacific, side of the country. The lowland Atlantic coastal area was relatively protected from both the Somoza repression and the hardships of the insurrection. As will be discussed in the next chapter, the very different geographies, histories, and cultural backgrounds of the peoples of the Eastern and Western Coasts would later be reflected in the different models of primary health care in the two areas after the Sandinista victory.

PRIORITIES FOR RECONSTRUCTION

Despite the extensive damage done to health facilities during the insurrection, and the fact that the Sandinistas moved quickly to establish the National Unified Health System, three other priorities outranked health on the government's agenda. A crucial insight into the dynamics at work, though, is to see the interelatedness and interdependence between the priorities.

Defense of the revolution was placed above all other priorities. To implement the necessary structural changes, a strong defense against contrary interests, both domestic and international, was required. Toward this end the Sandinistas organized a civilian militia which, after four years, numbered 60,000 men and women (Walker 1984:8). In 1983, a compulsory military draft was instituted.

The second priority for the Sandinistas was economic: price supports for basic commodities; increase in the production of export crops; refinancing of the national debt; and agrarian reform. Workers of the one million hectares of former Somoza family lands (20 percent of Nicaragua's total arable land) were organized into cooperatives and state production units (UPEs). By 1982, more than 40,000 landless rural families had received access to land on which to grow their own food, and prerevolutionary levels of production were surpassed in all basic food crops (Collins 1982:4,152). The changes made in the economy have had an important impact on health inasmuch as nutritional levels are directly affected by food production and distribution as well as by the ability of the population to purchase staples.

The third priority was education. As with defense and the

economy, education has important implications for health status. The illiteracy rate in Nicaragua prior to the Revolution was 50.3 percent and school enrollments stood at about 501,000. In 1980, the Government trained 100,000 literacy workers to travel into the countryside and teach the peasants. By 1981 the illiteracy rate had reportedly dropped to 12.9 percent. By 1982 some 613,000 persons had been taught to read and write and school enrollments have doubled to over 1,000,000 (Assmann 1981; Miller 1985).

The fourth priority, as stated, was health. The National Unified Health System (SNUS) brought together twenty-three semiautonomous bureacracies that had duplicated and fragmented health services before the revolution. This consolidation was precisely what had been recommended by USAID in the Chinandega reform of 1976 (Chapter 2). The Sandinistas went further and declared health to be a public good for which the State and the people shared mutual responsibility. Six principles were to be the basis of health organization.

1. Health is a right of every individual and a responsibility of the State and the Popular Organizations.

2. Health services ought to be accessible to the entire population, geographically, economically and culturally.

3. Health services should function to integrate the physical, mental and social dimensions of health and to address the conditions of work and residence as they affect health.

4. Health care ought to be delivered in a multi-professional team effort.

5. Health activities are to be planned.

6. The community ought to participate in all activities of the health system (MINSA 1981b:17-21).

BUILDING POPULAR PARTICIPATION IN HEALTH PLANNING

In the late stages of the insurrection, access to health facilites was severely restricted by the fighting and the intimidation of the National Guard. As a result, many physicians and nurses went into the barrios and trained people to provide emergency care to both combatants and civilians. Some physicians supplied medicines from hospital stores to a clandestine network of mobile clinics and pharmacies. Others trained members of the neighborhood Civil Defense Committees (CDCs) to perform emergency surgery. CDCs were instructed on how to dispose of corpses so as to minimize health hazards. Emergency plans were developed in the neighborhoods in the event that water supplies became affected or were cut off.

There emerged from this experience a cadre of health workers who had first-hand training in health care and sanitation. After the insurrection, some of the same people became the Health Coordinators (Responsables de Salud) in the neighborhood Sandinista Defense Committees (CDSs). In September and October of 1979 an antipolio and antirabies vaccination campaign was carried out in which the CDS Health Coordinators actively participated.

The insurrection itself was a primer in local organization for health whose impact was soon to be felt in the Sandinista health programs at the levels of planning, organization and delivery of services.

The health planning function in National Unified Health System provided for the inclusion within the Ministry of Health of several different constituencies and points of view on health delivery. In addition to the physicians who generally represent a medical and institutional perspective, the planning function also involves the Division of Communication and Popular Education in Health ("Division de Comunicacion y Educacion Popular en Salud" DECOPS) created in March 1980. These health educators tend to define health in social as well as biological terms and stress a more popular and preventive strategy rather than an institutional and curative one. This office would become the major advocate for a popular health care model within the health bureauracy. Its first task was to prepare between March and August 1980 some 200,000 copies of "Health Lessons for Literacy Workers" and train 12,325 literacy workers in malaria prevention and treatment. During 1981 some 224 Oral Rehydration Units were organized around the country for the prevention and control of diarrhea in children (MIPLAN/MINSA 1981:7).

Health planning has been given both a professional and a public forum. The analysis and summary workshops ("jornadas de analysis y balance" JABs) are regular meetings held at the regional and national levels. Health professionals meet to discuss previously set health objectives, performance, and continuing needs. Discussions evolve around why objectives have or have not been met and corrective strategies are agreed upon. The first JAB was held in 1979 after some months of experience in meeting the health needs of the population immediately after the Revolution. One result of that effort was the decision to decentralize the health bureauracy. The Emergency Plan of 1980 called for the creation of nine health regions and within each region the creation of health areas (MINSA 1981b:79). The Health Regions were redefined in May 1982 to conform to the National Plan of Regionalization, which brought all government agencies under the same regional jurisdictions. The new alignment resulted in six health regions and three special zones on the Altantic Coast (see Figure 3.1).

POPULAR ORGANIZATIONS

The decision, made in 1980 to have DECOPS form popular health councils ("consejos populares de salud" CPSs) at local, regional and national levels, further enhanced popular participation in a public forum. The creation of popular health councils as well as face-the-people meetings between government officials and people ("cara al pueblo") provided for direct input by the popular organizations and by the local community into the health planning and evaluation process. Before turning to an analysis of the impact of these various bodies on the planning process, a more detailed description of the popular organizations and their experience in health delivery is in order.

The Sandinista government organized the population into associations, called mass organizations ("organizaciones de masas"), each of which would participate in activities related to the four priority areas of defense, the economy, education, and health. The most active organizations in the health sector have been the Sandinista Defense Committee (CDSs) and The Luisa Amanda Espinoza National Association of Nicaraguan Women ("Asociacion de Mujeres Nicaraguenses 'Luisa Amanda Espinoza'" AMNLAE). The CDSs has a geographical constituency on the neighborhood or rural sector level, and AMNLAE focuses its concerns directly on how women might contribute to the revolutionary process.

Other organizations have occupational memberships, such as the Federation of Health Workers (FETSALUD), the Confederation of Sandinista Workers (CST), the National

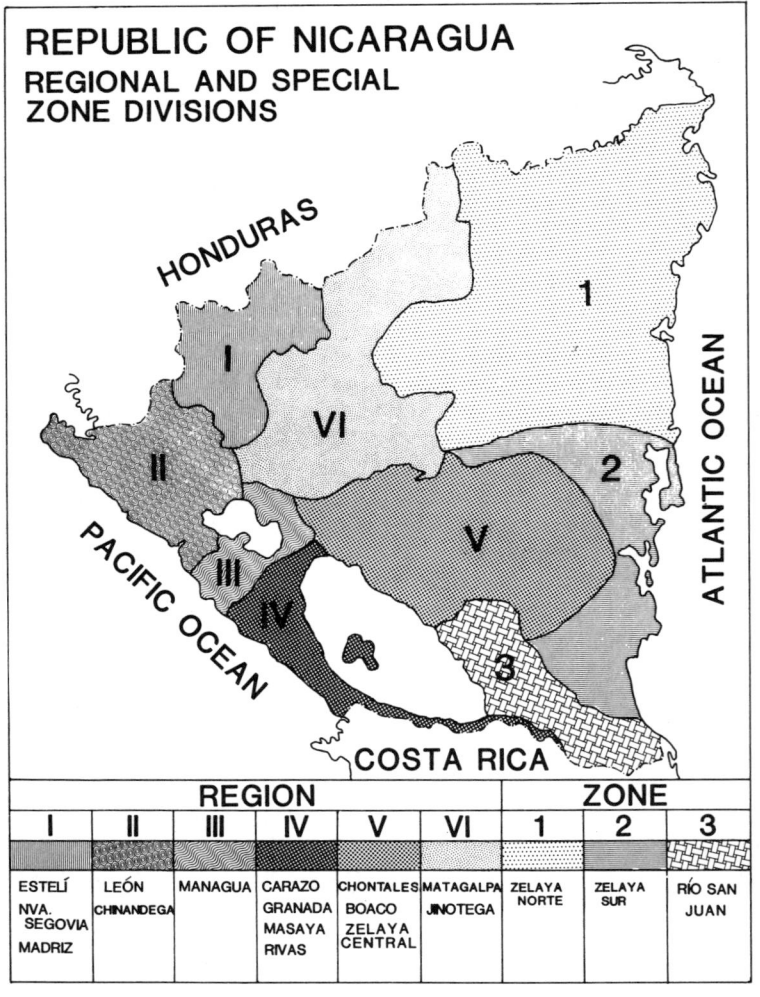

FIGURE 3.1

Association of Nicaraguan Educators (ANDEN), and the Association of Agricultural Workers (ATC). The Sandinista Youth "19th of July" (JS19J) and the Sandinista Children's Association (ANS) incorporate children and young people into the reform programs. The Parent's Association (APF) addresses educational and other familial matters. Figure 3.2 illustrates the organization of participation in health within these popular health councils.

HEALTH DELIVERY: A QUESTION OF CONTROL

In 1980 the Ministry of Health and the Popular Health Councils agreed to organize several mass drug administration and sanitation campaigns at the national level (Garfield and Taboada 1984). These were called popular health work days ("jornadas populares de salud" JPSs). The idea had emerged from successful organizing efforts in health care during and immediately after the insurrection. The Government viewed the health days as an opportunity to focus the attention of governmental bodies and popular organizations on a common activity. It was felt that this experience would serve as a model for organizing grass-roots activities in areas other than health.

Major organizational responsibility for the health days resided in the Divison of Education and Popular Communication in Health and the popular health councils (CPSs) organized earlier that year. DECOPS originally had intended the health councils to be made up exclusively of the popular organizations. They could thereby better negotiate community health concerns and strategies with the Ministry as a partner in planning. However, with the emergence of the popular health days in 1981, the health councils became a joint body of representatives from the popular organizations and the Ministry. The effect was to dilute the independent planning and evaluation function of the popular organizations within the health councils. The councils were subordinated to the centralized planning of the Ministry while the popular organizations were more involved in the execution stages of the health work days (Keyzer and Ulate 1980:133).

The health days provided the first indication that two competing philosophies of primary health care delivery existed within the Ministry, and that some resolution of this competition would eventually be necessary (DECOPS/MINSA 1982:1); see Chapter 5.

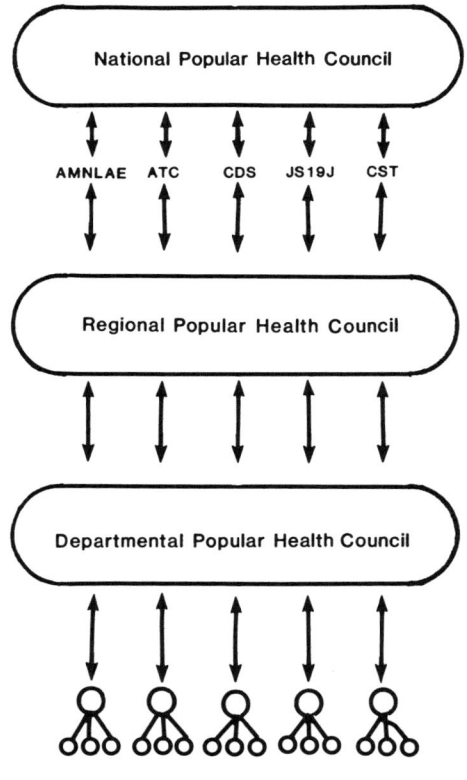

Figure 3.2. Structure of Popular Participation in Health in Nicaragua

Four national popular health campaigns were carried out in 1981. These included an antipolio campaign in two phases, an environmental sanitation campaign, an antidengue campaign, and the most ambitious of the four, an antimalaria campaign (Garfield and Vermund 1983b). In 1982, the popular health days continued at the national level. In November and December of that year there began a national effort to train 8000 primary health care workers ("brigadistas de atencion primaria" BAPs) in the basic concepts of primary health care for mothers and children and first aid. Table 3.1 illustrates the extent of the early organizational efforts. Table 3.2 and Figure 3.3 indicate the number of persons vaccinated and doses provided over a four year period. The impact of the vaccination program can be observed in Table 3.3 and Figure 3.4 which report the number of cases and morbidity rates for five common childhood diseases.

The popular health days raised several questions about the lack of coordination between the Ministry and the popular organizations. The Ministry of Health was organized into nine health regions and into clinic areas within each region. This organizational structure did not always conform to that of the popular organizations, which were structured along county ("municipio") and state ("departamento") lines. An organizational compromise was effected in which logistic support for the health days would be provided at the area clinic level, while programing and promotion would be coordinated at the municipal level. As a result of this experience, the government decreed in July 1982 that all government agencies and Popular Organizations would have the same regional structure and eventually the same municipal and area jurisdictions.

A second problem surfaced as a result of the experience of the health work days. The health days of 1981 and 1982 were planned centrally but carried out at the local level. This fact contributed to the perception of some among the popular organizations that the Ministry in Managua was ambivalent about sharing planning functions with them. In the words of one health worker, the Ministry considered itself "the lord and spokesman of the people." This conflict was illustrated during an upsurge of polio in 1981. Some within the Ministry called for "un Domingo Rojo y Negro" -- a "Red and Black Sunday" (1) on which the popular organizations would be asked to provide mass polio vaccinations. The Division of Popular Education and Commuication in Health resisted the suggestion to call up volunteers from the mass organizations on such short notice.

Table 3.1. Summary Statistics of the 1981 Popular Health Campaigns

	Antipolio First (March)	Antipolio Second (May)	Clean-up (June-July)	Antidengue (August)	Malaria (November)
Workshops	753	539	1269	1509	4062
Multipliers trained [a]	2170	2201	3716	8906	10,429
Brigadistas trained	17,687	15,073	19,755	77,619	73,594
Pamphlets distributed	500,000		1,200,000		
Vaccination posts	4911	4397			
Children vaccinated	341,975	301,160			
Persons medicated					1,892,746
Packages of Abate distributed [b]				1,000,000	
Tablets distributed [c]					35,000,000

Source: MINSA 1982c unpublished report. MINSA 1982d.
[a] Multipliers are volunteer health workers who in turn train Brigadistas
[b] Packages which contain an insecticide (temephos) that kills mosquito larvae
[c] Included 8 million packages of 25 million chloroquine and 10 million primaquine tablets

Table 3.2. Number of Persons Vaccinated and Doses Provided in Nicaragua for the Years 1980, 1981, 1982 and 1983

Type of Vaccine	1980[a]		1981[a]		1982[b]		1983[b]	
	Persons	Doses	Persons	Doses	Persons	Doses	Persons	Doses
B.C.G.	81,228	81,228	139,327	139,327	211,275	210,832	n/a	198,683
Polio	n/a	538,178	n/a	1,163,853[a]	n/a	1,489,707[c]	n/a	1,491,062
Measles	101,829	101,829	225,932[c]	225,932[c]	205,825[c]	205,323[c]	n/a	209,939
D.P.T.	n/a	384,949	n/a	410,693	n/a	880,480[c]	n/a	352,579
D.T.	46,817	156,411	56,722	155,229	85,088	236,745	n/a	202,721
T.T.	168,457	527,748	131,388	449,362	167,606	838,087	n/a	849,171
Total	n/a	1,790,343	n/a	2,544,396	n/a	3,859,174	n/a	3,304,155

Source:
[a] MINSA 1983:59,60, Tables 19 and 20.
[b] MINSA 1984:42-43, Table 3.
[c] Includes the activities of the Popular Health Work Days

34 The Nicaraguan Revolution in Health

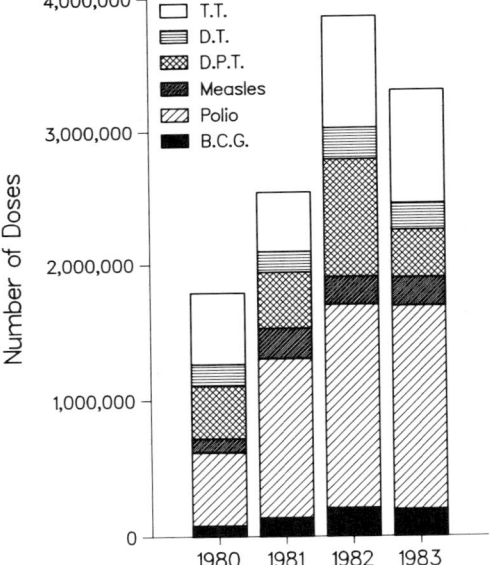

Figure 3.3 Number of Doses Provided in Nicaragua for the Years 1980, 1981, 1982 and 1983

Source: Table 3.2

Table 3.3. Transmittable Diseases Reported in Nicaragua and Rates per 100,000 Inhabitants 1980, 1981, 1982 and 1983

Disease	Number of Cases					Rate per 100,000				
	1980[a]	1981[a]	1982[b]	1983[b]	1984[c]	1980[a]	1981[a]	1982[b]	1983[b]	1984[d]
Poliomyelitis	21	46	0	0	0	0.7	1.6	0	0	0
Diphtheria	5	2	2	3	0	0.1	0.0	0.69	0.1	0
Whooping Cough	2,469	1,935	383	90	60	90.0	68.5	13.1	3.0	2
Tetanus	89	132	99	85	195	3.2	4.6	3.4	2.8	6.5
Measles	3,784	224	220	102	153	138.4	7.9	7.5	3.4	5.0

Source: [a] MINSA 1983:61, Table 21; [b] MINSA 1984:45, Table 3B; [c] MINSA 1985:24, Table 5; [d] my calculations

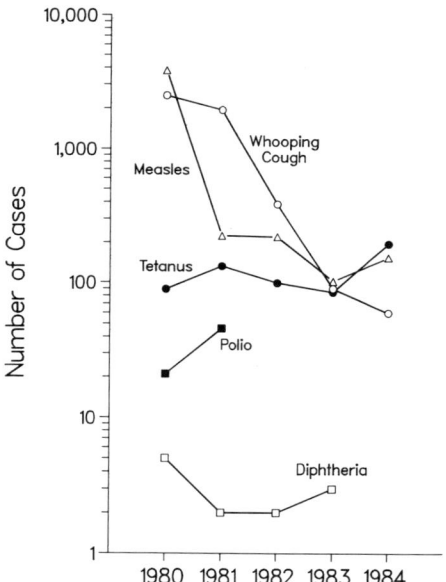

Figure 3.4. Cases of Transmittable Diseases Reported in Nicaragua 1980, 1981, 1982, 1983 and 1984

Source: Table 3.3

In addition, representatives from the popular organizations to the health councils were complaining that the Ministry physicians in the clinics were not meeting their health delivery goals. They interpreted the plan for another health day as a ploy to use volunteer "brigadistas" rather than demanding that the physicians be more resourceful themselves. Their objections prevailed and it was decided that efforts to provide polio vaccinations in the area clinics would be intensified. By 1983, the national health days were being replaced with regional health days. This decentralization corresponds in part to the demands of the popular organizations for more local control over planning. The policy change also reflected the fact that each region needed to adapt the health days to locally defined needs.

Popular vs Professional Control: A Case Study

The case study below illustrates conflicts between popular and professional agendas during the Popular Health Day on May 15, 1982. (2) The events took place in an urban center in Northern Nicaragua. The city is part of a Health Region organized into 17 Health Areas. Area "A" has 36 vaccination posts for some 5000 children in the urban sector and 30 posts for some 3000 rural children. A total of 334 people took part in the Health Day. Seventy were from the MINSA. The rest were members of the community and some medical students. All attended workshops prior to the health day in which procedures were discussed and assignments made. Each post had at least four people to meet and register patients. Although the publicity campaign was organized at the Municipal level, the local Sandinista Defense Committees (CDSs) were responsible for registration of children and for their health records. Each parent had an immunization card. A record of the vaccination was made on the card and on the registration sheet. If a child did not appear for the vaccination, the CDS personnel would visit the home to offer the vaccine or reschedule a sick child for a later appointment.

The supervisory team was made up of representatives of the Division of Popular Education and the Municipal Directors of the CDSs and AMNLAE. The team stopped in the Area Health Center and were promptly engaged by the physician. He complained that there had been no publicity in the neighborhood of the Health Center and reminded the supervisors that publicity was the responsibility of the MINSA. He commented that the downtown area was deluged with loudspeakers, but nothing happened in this neighborhood. He concluded that publicity for the JPSs might be better left to the local CDSs. The doctor went on to argue that the MINSA should provide each Health Brigadista with pencils and notebooks as well as a stipend for Saturday and Sunday work. Once outside, the team commented on the Doctor's observations. Since loudspeakers made their rounds in the neighborhoods early in the morning and in the evening (before and after Clinic hours), the Doctor was not around to hear them. They also remarked that MINSA-Managua had sent only $20,000 cordovas (US$2,000) for the JPSs in all the Region. Of that $11,000 cordovas went to the drivers for vehicle expenses. It would have been financially impossible to provide supplies and a stipend to the Health Brigadistas. More seriously such a policy of economic remuneration would have undermined the voluntary nature of the Health Work Days. Only the personal commitment of each Brigadista could make the JPSs economically feasible. As one team member concluded "Think of how much money it would cost if all these people were paid for their efforts."

The case reveals what may be more than a disagreement on procedures. The physician seemed to be projecting his entrepreneurial interests onto the Health Volunteers. More seriously his attitude may reflect a more fundamental conflict between popular organization for health and the traditional medical monopoly on health care. In that regard the JPSs are not the ultimate test of community participation in health.

In her study of popular participation in the health sector, Pechersky (1981) found that during 1981 most activity had been in the area of execution of programs, such as the JPSs. The JPSs were organized nationally and involved the local organizations less in planning and more in execution.

The real test of participation will be the extent to which the popular organizations can effect change within the local Health Centers and promote outreach activities. The acknowledged agendas of planning, programing, execution, supervision, evaluation, and development of new programs will be negotiated at the local level within the popular health councils. These interactions must be translated upwards through the departmental and regional councils to the national commission for an impact to be made on Ministry planning at the national level.

Popular Health Councils

It was noted earlier that DECOPS had major repsonsibility for the organization of the popular health councils (CPSs) at the local, departmental, regional, and national levels. This structural change within the National Unified Health System would add greater stature to populist participation strategies and their ability to compete with the advocates of professional control over health planning and service delivery.

Mention has already been made of the early change introduced into the CPS structure as a result of the decision to undertake national drug administration programs. To provide for greater coordination between governmental bodies and the popular organizations during the Popular Health Work Days, the Popular Health Councils became joint bodies of deliberation. This had the effect of concentrating local popular participation more on execution and less on planning and evaluation in the health sector. Another effect was to divert efforts away from the supervision of clinical personnel and the evaluation of health clinics and hospitals. These became more the issue in 1982 when the popular organizations turned their attention to the exercise of some control over health institutions and health personnel. To understand that change in focus, we now turn our attention to an analysis of the meetings of several CPS in northern Nicaragua. These meetings reveal the range of issues which the Popular Health Councils, as a participatory strategy, allowed to surface, be discussed, and acted upon. (3) The major themes include the structure and function of the CPS, brigadista training, supervision and evaluation of medical personnel and the coordination of the regional Popular Health Days. We will take up these four themes in order.

Not surprisingly several issues quickly surfaced when the CPS turned their attention to local issues of on-going health planning and delivery. The first was that of legal and moral accountability, often expressed in constitutions, by-laws, and standard operating procedures. When the CPS were created, the structure, composition, and hierarchy of the organization were spelled out only in a general way. The actual scope of the work and the operating procedures were devised at the municipal and departmental levels. In April 1982 (after about a year of operation) the Departmental CPS of El Arroyo voiced the need for written by-laws. Absenteeism on the part of the representatives from the CST (Sandinista Trade Union) and FETSAULD (The Federation of Health Workers) was high. FETSAULD was the focus of particular criticism for lack of interest. (This may have reflected the climate of criticism of health workers in the CPS.) Members noted that some of the mass organizations of the FSLN (The Sandinista Front of National Liberation) did not recognize the importance of the CPS. Members complained, for example, that the Departmental General Secretary of the FSLN in El Arroyo had called a Party Assembly during the last Popular Health Day. Participants called for closer collaboration with other state entities such as the National Peasant League (UNAC), the Agrarian Reform Agency (INDRA), and the National University (UNAM). On the other hand, the members argued that the ATC (Association of Peasant Workers), the CDS, and the CST (Confederation of Sandinista Workers) representatives on the CPS needed to provide more feedback from their bases. All agreed that each county district ("municipio") in the Department should have its own CPS and that a popular information network be created to link them together.

A second issue, which appeared in the meetings of the Departmental CPS of El Arroyo, was the relationship between professional personnel and the training of nonprofessional health brigadistas. There was agreement that brigadista training would include preventive medicine, vital statistics, birthing and mother-child care as well as occupational health care. The program, designed for the rural areas, would first be piloted in an urban neighborhood. Medical personnel from the area clinic would provide the training.

Brigadista selection would be made on the basis of a profile jointly developed by the CDS, AMNLAE (The Nicaraguan Women's Association), and The Ministry of Health. All agreed that Health brigadistas should be designated as such, so that their health responsibilities not conflict with other tasks. (The latter observation seems to have been precipitated by the fact that some volunteers entered the training program as a way to fulfill service prerequisites for FSLN Party membership. As noted earlier, Party obligations, such as attendance at Assemblies, could compete with the health tasks of the volunteers.)

A third, and potentially the most sensitive of the issues raised in the CPS meetings, was the evaluation and supervision of medical personnel in the area clinics and hospitals. The CPS requested that the MINSA advise it when evaluations were to be held. They stipulated that health personnel be evaluated on their performance in the areas of preventive medicine and popular education. One area clinic was singled out for specific criticisms. Members pointed out that physicians were not keeping their hours in the area clinic of El Carmen. Patients were often treated condescendingly. To provide more accountability in provider-patient relationships, the CPS agreed to recommend that all health personnel wear a name tag for easier identification. Another complaint was that some people were made to wait in line while others were brought forward because of favoritism ("el amiguismo"). The CPS asked that the clinic look for more efficient ways to handle the patient load. They recommended increased use of volunteers in clerical tasks. Another criticism of the care at El Carmen clinic dealt with acute care and quality of service. Eye and hand lacerations were not treated as emergencies and referrals to specialists took up to three months. (The reference was to sugar cane workers who frequently suffer from lacerations in the process of cutting and loading the stalks of cane.)

Another criticism was leveled at local hospital personnel in El Arroyo who refused to accept expectant mothers who had not yet dilated 5 centimeters. The CPS argued that the inflexible application of that norm was not in tune with the felt needs of the patients. The CPS recommended that the Directors of the Area Clinics meet with the Director of the hospital to seek ways to improve the quality of obstetric care and the better utilization of the obstetrics ward.

Another series of deliberations dealt with the role of folk healers ("los curanderos") in health care. The CPS in the nearby rural distict of Rio Viejo had asked the Regional Office of MINSA to name the local curandero to their newly constructed health post. At the same time, the MINSA had ordered a curandero in another village to stop practicing medicine there. The people from that village had written to La Barricada, the national newspaper of the Sandinista Party, and complained. The Departmental CPS in El Arroyo responded by commissioning AMNLAE to take a census of all practitioners of folk medicine ("los recursos empiricos") in the Department. These events seem to have precipitated a special meeting of the Popular Organizations and the MINSA in El Arroyo on April 12, 1982. The objective of the meeting was to elaborate a general policy towards curanderos. The meeting had the effect of putting further action by the MINSA on hold. In fact, the discussion of curanderos revealed common complaints against the professional practitioners of medicine. The curandero is available day and night; the physician only during the day... The curandero makes home visits while the physician never moves from the clinic... The curandero is a confidant and gives emotional support to the patient...The curanderos practice of medicine is more in accord with the beliefs and expectations of the people... The curandero shares his knowledge, but the doctor does not explain or educate one to the nature of the illness or the reason for the treatment... The people can tell the difference between the illnesses which a curandero can treat and those he cannot, but people often go only to them because professional health services are not available...

The significance of the CPS, as a participatory strategy, is that it created within the health sector a forum for a constituency other than that of the professionals. Yet, the issue of professional control did not go away. Since the Health Work Days were first organized in 1981, the health professionals have been able to exercise their cultural and social authority within the CPS. This authority now seems to be challenged more as the CPS turn their attention to the institutional aspects of health care. The conflict of professional/populist agendas would emerge again in the area of formal Brigadista training and will be discussed at length in Chapter 5.

The Ministry of Health

The experience of the popular organizations in health in the first eighteen months of the revolution coincided with a second and quite different focus within the MINSA. Although the popular organizations were engaged in massive vaccination campaigns, popular health education programs, and other preventive strategies, much of the institutional support within the MINSA was going to the reconstruction of hospitals and the construction of new primary care clinics. Primary care efforts focused upon the expansion of out-patient clinic services and the preparation of volunteer health workers ("brigadistas de atencion primaria" BAPs) who would work under the supervision of the Clinic Director and the Area Nurses. (4)

By mid-1980, however, the popular health constituency within the MINSA and in the Popular Health Councils were able to challenge the more institutional approach to primary care. The Neuro-Surgeon Minister of Health was replaced by a member of the Sandinista leadership, Lea Guido, who was not a physician. The change in Ministry leadership signaled a new policy direction in the health sector more in keeping with the Government's own efforts to contain costs. The Government of Reconstruction initiated in 1981 the National Austerity and Efficiency Plan. This change in national policy and Ministry of Health leadership allowed DECOPS and the popular organizations to argue for a more popular, broad-based and cost-effective approach to primary health care. The result was that new hospital and clinic construction program begun in 1980 was curtailed in 1981. (New clinic and health post construction would resume in 1982, as discussed below.) While financial constraints in 1981 favored a cost-effective primary care model, the fact that DECOPS and the popular organizations had already successfully trained health workers and organized thousands of Nicaraguans in vaccination and malaria campaigns provided credibility to their strategy. At the same time, WHO and UNICEF offered technical and financial assistance to expand the Primary Care Program and the training of health workers throughout the country (UNICEF 1983).

IMPACT OF THE NEW HEALTH PROGRAM

The impact of the health policy changes initiated by the Revolution and carried forward during the first several years of the Revolution are visible in the changing profile of medical care and epidemiological indicators. (5)

Accessibility of Medical Care

One of the principles of the National Unified Health System is to make health care more accessible to everyone, and a priority of the MINSA has been to provide more service to the medically underserved areas of the country and to increase medical encounters. The number of medical encounters has doubled since 1977, and the most significant increases have occurred in those areas of greatest need: Region I (Esteli), Region V (Chontales, Boaco), Region VI (Matagalpa, Jinotega), and in the special zones of the Atlantic Coast (see Map 3.1, Table 3.4 and Figure 3.5). Managua (Region III) continues to lead the country in medical encounters, although there was a slight drop in 1982. Indeed, Managua's share of the total medical encounters of the country decreased from 64 percent in 1977

Table 3.4. Number of Medical Encounters[a] in Nicaragua by Health Region and Special Zone for the Years 1977, 1980, 1981, 1982 and 1983[d]

Regions and Special Zones	Number of Medical Encounters				Encounters per Inhabitant			
	1977	1980	1981	1982	1977	1980	1981	1982
National	2,432,925	4,982,623	5,411,432	6,022,634	1.0	1.8	1.9	2.1
I	56,882	387,622	484,772	597,671	0.2	1.4	1.7	2.0
II	372,758	713,122	655,725	765,904	0.9	1.5	1.4	1.6
III	1,565,820	2,201,115	2,353,420	2,291,777	2.1	2.8	2.9	2.7
IV	197,742	820,800	864,157	917,090	0.5	1.7	1.8	1.8
V	42,459[b]	347,573	291,298	351,583	0.2	1.4	1.1	1.3
VI	80,391	233,556	446,631	598,395	0.3	0.7	1.3	1.7
S-Z 1	116,873[c]	132,884	145,992	295,062	0.9	1.8	1.9	3.7
2	–	140,028	163,196	175,077	–	2.6	2.9	2.9
3	–	5,923	6,241	30,075	–	0.2	0.2	1.0

ce: MINSA 1983:28, Table 2.

[a] Includes encounters in hospitals and area health clinics
[b] Includes Special Zone 3
[c] Includes Special Zones 1 and 2
[d] Only national totals were published for 1983. They included 6,467,187 medical encoutners or 2.14 encounters per inhabitant (MINSA 1984:40, Table 1).

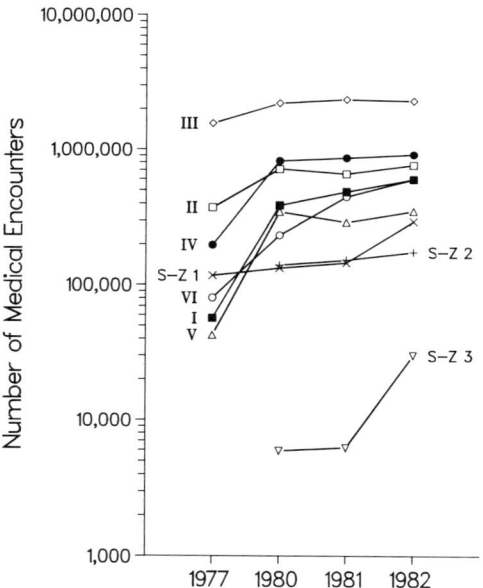

Figure 3.5. Number of Medical Encounters in Nicaragua by Health Region and Special Zone for the Years 1977, 1980, 1981, and 1982

Source: Table 3.4.

to 38 percent in 1982. This may reflect the redistribution of medical personnel to more underserved areas of the country (see Table 3.5 and Figure 3.6).

There is a concern with the quality of care in this rapid expansion of medical encounters. There is no universally accepted triage system in the area clinics; whoever walks in the door will see a physician. This policy is not a cost-effective use of professional resources, but it seems to be deliberate. The popular health councils may support the policy because of people's preference for seeing physicians and obtaining prescriptions. The policy also reaffirms the medical model of healing and physician control over health care. The policy might therefore reflect a convergence of professional and patient interests. Clinics are crowded, and many physicians seem overwhelmed by the patient load. In some cases encounters are perfunctory, and since no one will be turned away on a given day, there is no incentive for patients to schedule appointments. Nor are physicians guaranteed that they will have a minimum amount of time to see each patient.

Hospital and Clinic Facilities

Hospital construction has barely kept up with the growth of population. In 1977, there were 588 persons per available hospital bed as compared to 598 persons per available bed in 1984 (see Table 3.6). In 1980, the number of hospital beds had increased by more than 300 over the number available in 1977. After the revolution, the MINSA took over operation of three private hospitals. Meanwhile, there was a redistribution of hospital bed capacity in an attempt to achieve greater equity in the allocation of those scarce resources (see Table 3.7 and Figure 3.7). The greatest increases in the number of hospital beds between 1977 and 1982 are to be found in the the most underserved regions of Esteli/ Nueva Segovia (I), Rivas (IV), Chontales/Boaco (V), and Zelaya Norte (Special Zone 1).

During 1981 and 1982, several hospitals were closed as an economy measure. The net increase in available beds over the next two years was only 88, as hospital construction already under way fell behind schedule and new construction was constricted (see Table 3.7). A new hospital is being built by the Soviets in Chinandega to replace the one destroyed in the May 1982 floods, and four other large clinics with added inpatient care are underway.

The slowing of hospital construction is paralleled by a

Table 3.5. Distribution of Physicians[a] in Nicaragua by Health Region and Special Zones for the Years 1980, 1982[c] and 1983[d]

Region and Special Zone	No. of Physicians per 10,000 Inhabitants	
	1980	1982
I	1.98	2.86
II	3.93	4.37
III	7.0	7.9
IV	3.3	4.7
V	1.17	3.5
VI	2.0	3.42
S-Z 1	[e]	8.2
S-Z 2	2.2	5.1
S-Z 3	5.7	[f]
National	4.4	5.24

Source: MINSA 1981b:87; 1983:89, Table 31.

[a] Figures include only Nicaraguan physicians
[b] The 1980 total of 1212 physicians includes 34 assigned to administrative duties.
[c] The 1982 total of 1541 physicians includes 34 assigned to administrative duties.
[d] A total of 1,593 physicians were in practice in 1983 and 1.474 in 1984. Another 747 physicians were from other countries (MINSA 1984:104, Table 21; 1985:27, Table 27). Regional distributions were not available.
[e] Included in Region V
[f] Included in Region V

48 The Nicaraguan Revolution in Health

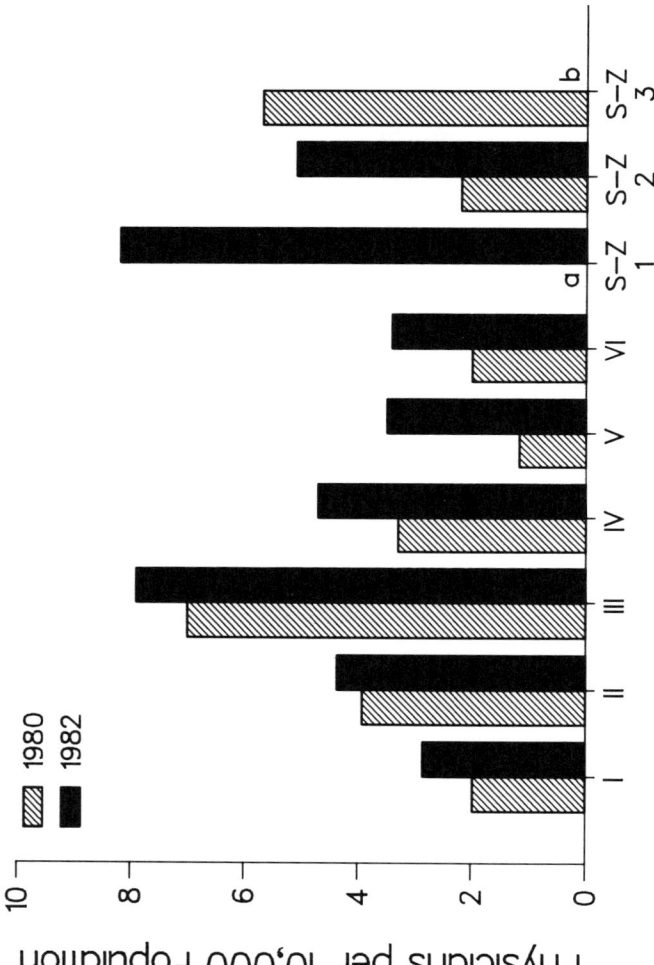

Figure 3.6. Distribution of Physicians in Nicaragua by Health Region and Special Zones for the Years 1980 and 1982

Source: Table 3.5.

Table 3.6. Hospital Capacity and Usuage in Nicaragua 1977,1980,1981,1982[a],1983[b], 1984[c]

Year	Number of Beds	Population /Available Bed	Number of Discharges	Number of Discharges /100 Pop.
1977	4313	588	120,952	4.8
1980	4677	588	178,017	6.5
1981	4729	625	190,577	6.7
1982[d]	4765	625	197,214	6.8
1983	n/a	n/a	211,382	7.0
1984[d]	5040	598	200,878	6.7

Source: [a]MINSA 1983:80,82, Tables 26 & 28.
[b]MINSA 1984:40, Table 1.
[c]MINSA 1985:23, Table 2.
[d]Includes acute and chronic care hospitals and health centers with beds for all years.

Table 3.7. Hospital Bed Capacity[a] in Nicaragua 1977, 1980, 1981, 1982 and 1984

Health Region/ Special Zone	Number of Beds					Change		
	1977	1980	1981	1982	1984	77&82(b)	80&82(c)	82&84(d)
I	298	420	388	392	375	+94	-28	-17
II	882	752	784	844	853	-38	+92	+9
III	1561	1687	1639	1607	1598	+46	-80	-9
IV	699	733	750	790	821	+91	+57	+31
V	185	279	289	294	247	+109	+15	-47
VI	512	471	498	508	461	-4	+37	-47
1	47	127	168	133	69	+86	+6	-64
2	129	157	153	130	132	+1	-27	+2
3	e	51	60	67	67	n/a	+16	0
National Totals	4313	4677	4729	4765	4623	+385	+88	-140

Source: MINSA 1983:80, Table 26; 1985:23, Table 1.

[a] Includes acute and chronic care hospitals and health centers with beds.
[b] The difference in the number of beds between 1977 and 1982.
[c] The difference in the number of beds between 1980 and 1982
[d] The difference in the number of beds between 1982 and 1984.
[e] Included in Region V

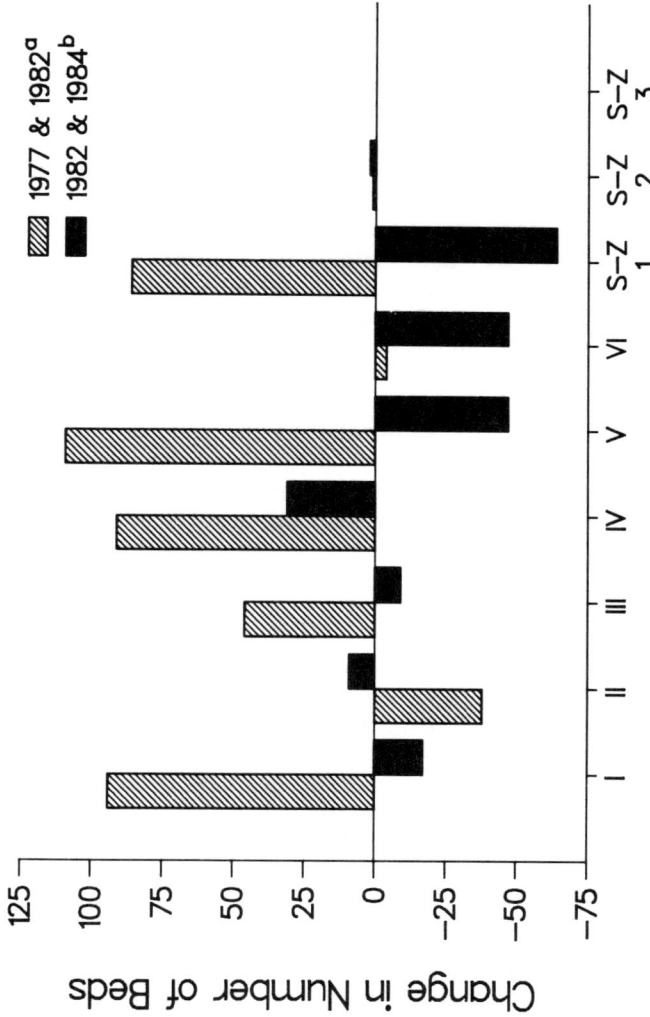

Figure 3.7. Changes in Hospital Bed Capacity in Nicaragua 1977 and 1982, 1982 and 1984

Source: Table 3.7.

[a] see note b, Table 3.7.
[b] see note d, Table 3.7.

decrease in the number of surgical procedures performed in the country. The number of surgeries increased from 36,052 in 1977 to 54,457 in 1980, in part because of the large number of war casualties. The number remained virtually unchanged in 1981 and 1982, and in fact, the number of surgeries per 100 people declined from 1.99 in 1980 to 1.87 in 1982 (MINSA 1983:81, Table 27). It may be that the demand for surgical procedures declined once the wartime causalties were cared for. The poor distribution of surgeons in the country, combined with deteriorating equipment and lack of supplies, has also contributed to the decline. As a result, some patients have been sent overseas for needed surgery. As inpatient hospital bed capacity stabilized, there was an increase in hospital usage as measured by the number of discharges (see Table 3.6). On the other hand, a comparison of medical encounters in outpatient clinics and hospitals indicates that there are three medical encounters in primary care facilities for every one in a hospital (see Table 3.8). In fact, in 1980 and 1981, one can note what may represent a gradual shift in medical encounters from hospitals to community health centers. (The decrease in clinic and health post encounters in 1981 may reflect the building moratorium in that year.) (6) The decrease in hospital encounters may be due to an increase in the number of health centers and posts and to more effective care at the local level (see Table 3.9). The 1982 total of 453 health clinics and posts represents a 24 percent increase over the 366 built in the first eighteen months of the revolution and almost a 200 percent increase over the 115 in existence in 1975 (USAID 1976:91).

After the flurry of construction in 1980, only seven new health clinics and posts were opened in 1981. Another 80 were built in 1982, and twenty-six were reconditioned. Rural areas in Regions I, II, III, IV, and Special Zone 1 benefited from most of the health clinic expansion in 1982. Increased contra (7) attacks in 1983 and 1984 resulted in the destruction of four clinics in Region VI (Matagalpa/ Jinotega). A total of 140 beds were lost, many because of contra activity (see Table 3.7).

The expansion of dental services parallels the establishment of primary care facilities during the same period (see Table 3.10). The major expansion of dental services between 1977 and 1982 occurred in Region V (Chontales and Boaco) and Region VI (Matagalpa and Jinotega), which registered an increase of over 400 percent (MINSA 1983:34 Table 7).

The above analysis suggests that health care, as

Table 3.8. Medical Encounters in Nicaragua in Health Centers and Hospitals 1980, 1981, 1982 and 1983

Medical Encounters

Type of Facility	1980[a] No. (%)	1981[a] No. (%)	1982[b] No. (%)	1983[b] No. (%)
Health Center and Post	3,013,824 (60.5)	3,039,595 (57.2)	3,853,874 (64)	4,243,125 (66)
Hospital	1,968,799 (39.5)	2,317,837 (42.8)	2,180,571 (36)	2,224,062 (34)
Total	4,982,623 (100)	5,411,432 (100)	6,034,445 (100)	6,467,187 (100)

Source: [a]MINSA 1983:28-30, Tables 2, 3, and 4.
[b]MINSA 1984:40-43, Tables 1, 2, and 3.

Table 3.9. Health Clinics and Health Posts in Nicaragua by Health Regions and Special Zones for the Years 1980, 1981, and 1982

Variables	Year	National Level	Regions and Special Zones								
			I	II	III	IV	V	VI	1	2	3
Number of Units	1980	366	40	67	42	71	75	43	13	15	a
	1981	373	40	67	44	71	75	47	14	15	a
	1982	453	54	80	62	85	79	40	24	15	14
	1984	487	55	89	75	87	87	43	22	14	15
Number of Units per 10,000 Population	1980	1.3	1.4	1.5	0.5	1.5	2.6	1.3	1.8	2.8	a
	1981	1.3	1.4	1.4	0.5	1.5	2.6	1.4	1.8	2.7	a
	1982	1.5	1.8	1.6	0.7	1.7	3.0	1.1	3.0	2.5	4.6

Source: MINSA 1983:27, Table 1; 1985:23, Table 1.

[a] Data for Special Zone 3 appears in that of Region V for the years 1980–1981.

Table 3.10. Dental Encounters in Nicaragua 1977, 1980, 1981, 1982, and 1983

Year	Dental Encounters	
	Number	Percent of Increase
1977[a]	203,540	—
1980[a]	258,742	27%
1981[a]	331,821	28%
1982[b]	417,078	26%
1983[b]	448,417	7%

Source: [a]MINSA 1983:34, Table 7
[b]MINSA 1984:42, Table 3.

measured by access to institutional care facilities, is much greater now than it was before the revolution. Policy changes that favored clinic over hospital construction greatly enhanced accessibility, and those changes reflect the participation of the popular organizations in the planning process both within the analysis and summary workshops (JABs) and the popular health councils (CPSs). The National Association of Nicargauan Women (AMNLAE) was especially active in the area of maternal-child care.

Maternal-Child Care

The expansion of clinics and hospitals has had a significant impact on children. Child medical encounters increased from 36 percent of total encounters in 1977 to 41 percent in 1982 (MINSA 1983:31,32 Tables 5 and 6), and much of the increase is due to maternal-child care programs. For instance, the number of pregnant women enrolled in the prenatal program rose from 82,599 in 1981 to 133,132 in 1982 (MINSA 1983:41, Table 9).

Between 1977 and 1982 the percentage of institutional births nationwide increased from 37 percent of all births to 43 percent (MINSA 1983:43 Table 11). Most of that increase took place in the first year of the revolution. Household and child care responsibilities, distance from hospitals, and the availability of local midwives may explain why many women may prefer home deliveries. In 1982, the MINSA organized a national board to formulate a policy for the selection and training of midwives. Several meetings were held, a training manual was published and training programs were piloted in Esteli and Leon/Chinandega. By mid-1983, more than 100 midwives had been trained and provided with birthing kits by UNICEF.

Postpartum care rose from 55,024 in 1981 to 111,288 in 1982, or from 67 percent to 84 percent of the participants in the prenatal care program (MINSA 1983:41, Table 9). By contrast, postpartum care in Special Zone 1 (Zelaya Norte) declined between 1981 and 1982 as the result of the increased hostilities along the Honduran-Nicaraguan border and the migration of the local population (MINSA 1983:42, Table 10).

A program to monitor child growth and development has widespread acceptance in the country, but underregistration of children affects estimates of the degree of coverage. Some 316,807 children participated in the program in 1982, up 80 percent from 176,072 in 1981 (MINSA 1983:52,Table 14).

An analysis of the program for malnourished children suggests that malnutrition will be an even more serious health problem as the Nicaraguan population continues to grow. In 1982, a total of 143,602 children were examined for nutritional deficiencies and provided with 148,826 follow-up examinations. Yet, this figure represents only 32 percent of possible beneficiaries. Of the total number of children examined in 1981 (72,904), 67 percent were classified as suffering from first-degree malnutrition (MINSA 1983:48), and the percentages of the prevalence of second- and third-degree malnutrition among Nicaraguan children ages zero to four years old for the periods of 1965-1967, 1974,1976, and 1981-1982 were 15.0, 22.6 and 34,0 percent, respectively (Teller 1981:11, MINSA 1983:53, Table 15). (8) An increasing birthrate will demand greater efforts to actually decrease the percentage of malnourished children in the population (Williams 1984:72-73). In 1980, a supplementary feeding program was initiated with the assistance of the World Food Program, and by the end of 1982, a total of 408,730 children and 76,808 pregnant women had participated in it.

In the first three years hospital deaths of children under the age of four due to diarrhea was reduced in the rankings from first to third place, partly because of the 330 oral rehydration units. It is hoped that this treatment will be given within the home and that mothers will be trained to utilize the salts on an early and routine basis (UNICEF 1983:1). Data indicate that utilization of the oral rehydration posts has begun to decrease in most regions (MINSA 1983:51, Table 13), and given the declines in hospital infant mortality, it may be that more mothers are now preparing the rehydration salts at home. Other public health measures taken since the revolution include environmental sanitation, rabies, tuberculosis, goiter, and malaria control programs.

Environmental Sanitation

Sanitation programs include potable water programs, liquid and solid waste disposal, school and work place sanitation. Water control activities included 1240 site inspections in 1981 and 1982 and 2509 water sample tests. By the end of 1982, 29,631 latrines have been installed (MINSA 1981b:55, 1983:66). In 1981-1982, waste disposal site inspections reached 7,697, garbage site inspections numbered 1,867, and garbage collection supervisions numbered

1,155. Food sanitation included 89,448 inspections of meat processing and packing plants, food processing plants, and food warehouses and distribution centers in that two-year period. Both environmental sanitation and rabies control programs received major support in the popular health work days carried out during those two years (MINSA 1983:58,75).

Tuberculosis Control

The tuberculosis program includes four elements: immunization, search for cases, treatment, and control of contagion. There were 81,228 childhood immunizations in 1980, 139,317 in 1981, and 211,275 in 1982. The ministry calculated that 2,817 new cases of TB would need to be treated in 1982, but only 1,330 were found. Of those, only 23 percent underwent the year-long treatment (MINSA 1983:56).

Malaria Control

The popular health day provided the organizational structure for a mass drug administration program in November of 1981 to control the transmission of malaria. The objective was to inhibit the transmission of the infection from humans to mosquitoes. If the infection could be eliminated in the general population for a period of three weeks, the mosquito could not acquire the malaria organism from human hosts and spread the infection. A three-day drug administration program was devised, and ʻa total of 25 million chloroquine and 10 million primaquine tablets were packages in 8 million color-coded envelopes of doses appropriate to each day and the age of the recipient (Garfield and Vermund 1983a:12). Popular participation was massive and it has been estimated that one in ten Nicaraguans was involved in promoting the campaign and disseminating information. Altogether, 70.1 percent (1,892,746) of the total population was treated (Garfield and Vermund 1983b:502). Monthly data collection showed that malaria incidence was considerably reduced for the four months following the campaign and that a total of 9,200 new cases of malaria were avoided (Garfield and Vermund 1983a:15). The total number of malaria cases in 1982 was 15,601, down from 17,434 in 1981 and 25,465 in 1980 (MINSA 1983:107, Table 31).

Goiter

Goiter was endemic in the country before the revolutiion (USAID 1976:189). Although no statistics are available on the current incidence of the disease, since 1980 the MINSA has supervised seventy-six salt mines, thirteen salt iodinization factories, and the wholesaling of iodized salt in the country.

A CASE STUDY: CHOROTEGA REVISTED

Impressive as the changes in health care have been, the statistics do not reveal the human struggle played out within the villages and neighborhoods around the country. To gain some insight into the process which underlie the improvements in health care, we return to Chorotega after the revolution.

Two years after the revolution the community of Chorotega can best be described as being in a period of transition. Changes are evident. A new dirt road runs from the highway to the village center. Electricity has reached the community. Some twenty men have formed a sisal cooperative to buy the material for hammocks at a cheaper price. Eight other men have formed a cattle cooperative. People indicated their pleasure with the fact that service and medicines at the hospital in town are free of charge. A private physician from another town periodically visits the community. Others remarked that the level of violence in the community had diminished substantially. Before the revolution a person arrested for assault or murder could buy his way out of jail. Today no guns are allowed in the commmunity and homocide brings a swift penalty of 30 years in jail.

In other respects Chorotega shows continuity with the past. There is a Sandinista Defense Committee (CDS) of eight members, the Central Coordinator of which is Don Jairo, the former Somoza political appointee (see Chapter 2). The former rural health coordinator (CRS) is now coordinator of the CDS for her area and is in charge of Popular Education for the Ministry of Education. As such, she supervises seven instructors who in turn are teaching adults in a followup program to the National Literacy Campaign. Her uncle is CDS coordinator for Economic Defense and Health.

The Popular Health Work Day (JPS) in Chorotega offers an

arena in which to observe the politics of change from the long tradition of vertical control to a more horizontal and democratic power base. Like many communities in Nicaragua, Chorotega is developing a political process less dependent upon patronage and corruption and more upon community participation in decision-making. This change is nowhere more evident than in the social arena of health delivery.

A Popular Health Day for polio and DPT was held in rural villages throughout Nicaragua on Sunday, May 16, 1982. There are 180 children five years and under registered in Chorotega. Yet, only 60 received DPT or polio vaccinations on that occasion. During the entire Sunday the evangelical sect remained in their chapel and would not participate in the vaccination program. One member (also CDS coordinator for Propaganda) indicated that one cannot serve two masters on the Lord's Day. Don Jairo also had called meetings of the evangelicals during the preparatory workshops for the JPS. His failure to participate in the JPS did not go unnoticed. The next day the Municipal Director of the CDS called the eight coordinators together. He strongly reprimanded Don Jairo's obstructionism.

Some community members feel that Don Jairo has co-opted the CDS and that his evangelism is a way to compete with the revolution. One community member indicated that Don Jairo maintains contact with a Somoza strongman in a nearby town and that his status of <u>Juez de Mesta</u> before the revolution went unchallenged when he was selected to be Center Coordinator of the CDS. People in the community may feel reluctant to challenge him for several reasons. A major one relates to Don Jairo's virtual monopoly on the local sale of sugar and basic food grains brought in from the town. The Sandinista government allows a markup to cover transportation costs, but Don Jairo seems to be making profit on dishonest weights and measures. It is a difficult charge to prove, but some community members were planning to take their purchases to the Sandinista Police in town to have the weight verified.

The case of Chorotega illustrates the two faces of politics and participation in Nicaragua: the patron-client brokerage role and the community role of accountability in the political process. That they exist side by side in Chorotega, or anywhere else, for that matter, should come as no surprise. What is different in Chorotega is that there is now in place a legitimate organization for community participation which can compete with traditional power brokers. Local accountability is now possible because their exists accountability at higher levels of government and vice versa. However, the challenge of any government is to find ways of institutionalizing the mechanism of accountability so that it does not depend on personal privilege or political orthodoxy. In health the sandinista defense committees and the popular health councils have proven to be two such mechanisms.

The process of health reform in Nicaragua since the revolution reveals several lessons about efforts of developing countries to provide "health to all by the year 2000." The first is that a government's political will to provide such care is essential. Comparisons of government efforts in public health before and after the revolution suggest significant differences in political commitment. The linkages between politics and health have been strong whenever countries with scarce resources have experienced rapid and significant improvements in the health of the general population, as in China (New and New 1975) and Cuba (Roemer 1976; Danielson 1979).

A second lesson is that once elimination of hunger and preventable diseases are made priorities, the state must organize its people for those tasks. Manpower and financial constraints make it impossible for health professionals and bureauracies to carry out those programs by themselves.

A third lesson is that once people are organized for massive public health programs, their organizational base will allow them to make further demands on the state for health care. Faced with scarce resources and the need to be cost-effective, the state must reconcile the institutional interests of those health professionals who practice in hospital settings and the demands of the organized people for a more broadly based and accessible primary care delivery system. The success of primary care delivery will depend on how much popular health organizations are able to participate in the health planning process. To be popular, participation must allow people, once organized, to initiate and formulate national and local health policies in ways that take them well beyond the tasks of implementation.

NOTES

[1] The colors of the flag of the Sandinista Liberation

Front are red and black. A "Red and Black Day" refers to a mobilization of popular organizations for a specific task.

[2] Names of places and of individuals have been changed to maintain anoymity.

[3] Data sources include interviews of participants and minutes of four meetings of two Departmental level CPS. The meetings were held between April and August of 1982. A fifth meeting on folk healers which took place on April 2, 1982 was between MINSA officials and representatives of the Popular Organizations. The place names have been changed to maintain anonymity.

[4] Primary health care is essential health care that includes education, promotion of basic food production and nutrition, potable water and sewage disposal, maternal and child care, immunizations, prevention and control of locally endemic diseases, simplified care of common diseases and injuries, and provision of essential drugs. Primary health care should be made universally accessible to individuals and families in the community by means acceptable to them, through their full participation and at a cost that the community and country can afford (WHO 1978:6).

[5] Where possible, data from the prerevolutionary period (pre-1979) has been included for comparative purposes. Data from the MINSA includes only public sector services.

[6] The use of medical encounters to compare health care delivery in hospitals and clinics understates the reality inasmuch as nursing encounters are not counted. Prenatal and postnatal care in the clinics as well as well-baby visits supervised by nurses are not reflected in the data. As a result, clinic activity is much greater than is suggested by medical encounters alone.

[7] The contras are a military force operating out of Honduras and Costa Rica, organized under the auspices of the Central Intelligence Agency. The officer corp is primarily composed of former members of the Somoza National Guard.

[8] Malnutrition, as measured by the Gomez classification, refers to the adequacy of a child's body weight as compared to the desirable standard for his or her age and sex. For example, second-degree malnutrition is 60-74 percent of the standard; third-degree malnutrition is below 60 percent.

Chapter 4
POPULAR EDUCATION IN HEALTH

The Sandinista Revolution of July 1979 set in motion a series of changes in the health delivery system that required mass popular participation. These changes included (1) the assignment of health roles to the Popular Organizations, (2) the preparation of Popular Organizations and volunteers to carry out mass vaccinations, and (3) the institution of Popular Health Commissions to coordinate activities between the Ministry of Health and the Popular Organizations. For the participation strategy to be effective, a redefinition of health education from the point of view of both content and pedagogy was required.

We now turn to an analysis of popular education in health in revolutionary Nicaragua since 1979. The intent is to look at the cultural and pedagogical underpinnings of popular education as reflected in a series of 17 Popular Health Pamphlets published in 1981 and seven Popular Health Documents published in 1981 and 1982. A content analysis will reveal how the Health Educators responsible for the elaboration of the documents attempted to combine in a culturally relevant manner the social and the biological components of primary health care and preventive medicine. We begin with a general statement of the issue addressed by "popular education" and the methodology involved. An illustrated analysis of the content and major themes found in the 24 Popular Health Pamphlets and Documents reveals how health education in Nicaragua conforms to the general goals and methodologies of popular education. (An illustrated summary of the content of each of the popular pamphlets is found in Appendix A.)

FRAMEWORK FOR POPULAR EDUCATION: FANON, FREIRE

To achieve the goal of a popular education for the largely illiterate populations of the Third World, Frantz Fanon (1963:151) proposed that language be used to empower people rather than control them from above.

> It is true that if care is taken to use only a language that is understood by graduates in law and economics, you can easily prove that the masses have to be managed from above. But if you speak the language of everyday, if you are not obsessed by the perverse desire to spread confusion and to rid youself of the people, then you will realize that the masses are quick to seize every shade of meaning and to learn all the tricks of the trade. If recourse is had to technical language, this signifies that it has been decided to consider the masses as uninitiated. Such a language is hard put to hide the lecturer's wish to cheat the people and to leave them out of things. The business of obscuring language is a mask behind which stands out the much greater business of plunder. The people's property and the people's sovereignty are to be stripped from them at one and the same time. Everything can be explained to the people, on the single condition that you really want them to understand.

Some 17 years later Commandant Tomas Borge would address the 100,000 Nicaraguan literacy workers as they began the National Literacy Crusade with these words:

> Those who are involved in the work of education ought to go with more than a book and an example. They ought to go to those places where organization needs to grow. We ought to put aside, therefore, every manifestation of paternalism and of elitism in order to understand what is necessary to lead the masses, but also to learn from the masses. We must have sufficient humility to understand that the people are full of wisdom and that they can teach us. This does not mean that we place ourselves at the level of backwardness of the most primitive sectors of the population, but that we begin

with that wisdom and learn from it so as to be able to educate.[quoted in MINSA 1980c; my translation]

The success of the National Literacy Campaign in reducing the rate of illiteracy from 50 percent to 13 percent was due to more than the goals of popular education voiced by Fanon and reiterated by Borge. In the intervening 17-year period there had emerged a pedagogy that has proven to be an effective means to carry out the task.

The Brazilian educator Paulo Freire wrote his book Pedagogy of the Oppressed in 1968. For Freire the purpose of education among the poor and illiterate people of the world is to humanize them as they learn to read and write. This means that education should free people from obstacles that impede their power of choice. For education to accomplish this task, it must make people aware of those obstacles. A society of self-determining people would be a truly free society.

Freire points out that the traditional "banking" style of education among the poor has often resulted in the reproduction of an unfree society within the following generation. By "banking," Freire refers to the process whereby the educator first identifies an object and then lectures his students about it. The object is "deposited" in the minds of the students through memorization (Freire 1970: 67-68). As such, traditional education prepares people to adjust to the status quo of a given society and to internalize alienating norms and values. Students are rewarded for their ability to memorize and repeat the "givens" of society. Banking education does not challenge students to examine critically the problematic nature of their social reality nor does it encourage them to take responsibility for improving the common good.

In contrast to the banking method of education, Freire presents "problem-posing education." To be humanizing, education must first change the relation of teacher-student from one of domination-subordination to one of cooperation and mutual respect. Second, the role of the teacher is not just to impart information, but to assist the students to problematize social reality. Third, Freire's method is characterized by dialogue in which teacher and students together analyze their reality with a mind to transform and improve it. In problem-posing education both teachers and students assume the responsibilty for the educational task. Both share the knowledge and experience which together provide the basis for the construction of a new society and not the simple reproduction of the old.

Problem-posing education is not merely an intellectual exercise antecedent to action. For Freire, action/reflection/action are inseparable components of an educational pedagogy in which knowledge is the power to create and transform. After several years' experience of popular education in the developing world, Freire concluded that problem-solving education must be tied to political action for the needed social transformations to take place. "So, the conclusion to which one arrives...", he states, "is that programs of popular education must be committed to a global strategy of action which among other things gives it meaning and directs its action" (Freire 1974:34, my translation). In other words, "popular education" for Freire is tantamount to "political education," not in a partisan sense, but in the sense that people can only create more humane conditions if they are able to organize themselves for political ends.

A corollary of this conclusion is that popular education embraces both formal and nonformal areas of educational endeavor. In either case the issue is how to design an educational system where the popular classes may act as the active and direct agents of their educational process. Freire concludes: "So, wherever the place may be, when distance is taken from the concrete context of a specific activity, we exercise a critical reflection on the action and in so doing have created a theoretical context, that is, a school, in the radical sense which this word should have" (quoted in Jara 1981:16, my translation and emphasis). The combination of action ("concrete context") and reflection ("theoretical context") in Freire's theory of learning is appropriate for education in institutional and noninstitutional settings. Such learning allows students to overcome the alienating character of that education which separates theory and action and intellect from morality. Furthermore, it is a concrete activity to improve the living conditions of the disenfranchised majority that links intellect amd morality. The critical analysis of reality is itself a pursuit of the truth whose goal is to free people from inhuman or less human conditions for more human conditions.

> Whereas banking education anesthetizes and inhibits creative power, problem-posing education involves a constant unveiling of reality. The former attempts to maintain the submersion of consciouness; the latter strives for the emergence of consciousness and critical intervention in reality. [Freire 1972:68]

Finally, Freire, like Fanon, argues that language is critical to motivate people to action and to give them the knowledge which empowers (1970:103ff). The choice of culturally relevant educational materials, the dialogue centered on concrete dimensions of social reality and popular organization are all predicated on one premise: knowledge is power. Whatever obfuscates, hides or distracts one from the reality under consideration is simply mystification. Popular education must seek to disseminate knowledge among the many, not concentrate it in the hands of the few; and it must lead to action and not to sterile debate.

THE NICARAGUAN PROGRAM

An early health education task facing the Ministry of Health was the preparation of the materials on public health to be incorporated into the National Literacy Crusade in March 1980. That experience demonstrated the need for materials and a methodology that would provide for massive dissemination of health information and knowledge. (1) In April 1980 the Division of Education and Popular Communication in Health was created within the Ministry, and Health Educators were assigned to each Health Center.

The First Seminar on Health Education was held in May 1980 with mixed results (MINSA 1981a:37). It was not until July and August that a clearer understanding of popular health education emerged. During a course for the Women's Association (AMNLAE) there was an effort to train health "multipliers" who in turn would form Health Brigadistas within the population at large. By September 1980 a philosophy of health education was materializing; it was set out in "Points of Departure for the Historical Analysis of Education and Popular Participation in Health" (MINSA 1980a) and in "Popular Education in Health: General Guidelines" (MINSA 1980c). During the Second National Seminar on Health Education in October 1980 the new methodology was developed further (2) and then presented to the Municipal Health Coordinators of the Sandinista Defense Committees. In essence, the new health education pedagogy envisions analysis of the structural as well as the individual roots of health and illness. Health education seeks to create the conditions, individual and social, which allow for the transformation of those structures. Popular education is defined as "a liberating process which permits the popular organizations to link the phenomenon health/illness to their historical and structural causes (interpreting these relations in a scientific manner) and to participate in decision-making, management and control of health programs, so as to transform their environment and better health conditions" (MINSA 1980a:42, my translation).

The educational philosophy underlying this pedagogy draws heavily upon the work of Freire.

> More important is the follow-up which we must give to the health workers ("responsables") once they are trained. We believe that the learning process is not just the transmission of knowledge, not the accumulation of information; rather, we believe that learning is the process which permits the acquisition, enrichment and dissemination of knowledge by way of a conscious and responsible action. By taking such an action an individual addresses the internal structure and the development of objective reality ("un objecto determinado") for the purpose of achieving its change or transformation. Learning as a dialectical process converts the student into an active agent, aware that objective reality must be faced with a political will. The student does not accept objective reality as having an immutable existence, but seeks to modify or transform it within the context in which he has been immersed. In this sense, knowledge, as a product of this process, is itself changing and growing day by day. As such, in the act of communication knowledge transcends the individual himself [MINSA 1980a:42, my translation].

In summary, the objectives of the Division of Popular Education are twofold: 1) They are to elevate the health educational level of the people; and 2) to provide them with the scientific knowledge necessary to develop activities and take collective actions that will help them solve their health problems. By contrast, in the traditional medical system, "only the physician possessed health concepts which conferred upon him power and prestige. The dominant ideology of the dictator made health a technological problem, isolated from the social context and, as such, from popular understanding.... Yet, the actual problem of health is not just a technical problem to be addressed only in the field of biology. It is also a social, economic and political problem... "(MINSA 1980a:39-40, my translation).

The process subscribed to by the Division of Popular Education is as follows: health education is to take place in the workshop where the Health Educator, Multiplier or Brigadista would lead the group in a dialogue that would have as its goal the demystification and popularization of health concepts ("la masificacion del conocimiento"); focus will be on the diagnosis of specific health problems and actions designed to solve them; workshops will be held for the popular organizations; the Popular Health Commission and Councils will provide a forum for on-going participation and evaluation.

To facilitate this process at the neighborhood level a series of Popular Health Pamphlets were produced and disseminated widely throughout the country prior to a specific Popular Health Campaign. All of these pamphlets were in a comic book design with cartoon figures and followed a standard format: A question on the cover introduces the pamphlet's content; a discussion guide is provided, followed by one or two "grand tour questions" on the topic to stimulate group dialogue. The group is encouraged to develop a response to the question before continuing with the reading of the pamphlet. After the reading, they are asked to compare their initial responses with what they had learned from the pamphlet. In addition to the 17 Popular Health Pamphlets published in 1981, eight Popular Health Documents were published for the more in-depth training of Health Multipliers and Brigadistas. They follow the same format, but are longer and incorporate more material than the Pamphlets (see Appendixes A and B).

HEALTH EDUCATION MATERIALS

Several considerations, based upon the experience of the National Literacy Crusade, were taken into account in the preparation of the teaching materials. Educational materials do not themselves insure learning. Learning is enhanced by the discussion of the materials. They must be so prepared so as to stimulate dialogue. Most of the pamphlets begin with a "Guide," which directs the participants to begin by analyzing the initial questions. This first step in the dialogue is referred to as "decodification" (Freire 1970:114; Jara 1981:52). The questions refer the participants to an illustration. They are asked to describe the situation presented in the picture. The picture contains one or more "generative themes" or representations of the concepts, values, and obstacles that impede the solution of a particular health problem. The "picture code" is split apart and analyzed to extract the implicit themes and their connections. The purpose of the decoding is to pose a problem in such a way that the participants can identify the themes implicit in the visual code.

A case in point is the pamphlet entitled "The Causes of Diarrhea ..." in which the group is asked to link the two generative themes of "diarrhea" and "living conditions" (Figure 4.1). The study guide begins with an analysis of how and why class differences affect the incidence of diarrhea among children. In this case the themes of illness and living conditions are linked to observed inequalities in income. The questions elicit the objective as well as the subjective or native understanding of their reality.

Children whose parents enjoy good living conditions are less susceptible to diarrhea. Yet, diarrhea is the most common illness in Nicaragua and the one which causes most deaths to children under six years of age. The Revolution seeks to provide all Nicaraguans with access to the basic living conditions which encompass the work place, food, housing, a clean environment, education and health services.

After the initial decoding, each pamphlet guides the participants through a discussion of the personal and structural causes of illness, be they social, cultural, economic or political in nature. In the pamphlet on diarrhea, an illness of children is attributed to a socioeconomic cause, the inequities in the distribution of wealth. These inequities are being addressed by the Revolution, some of whose effects can already be seen (Figure 4.2).

The cultural roots of illness is another theme coded in the pamphlets. Examples of this theme can be found in the analysis of beliefs ("creencias") regarding breastfeeding (Figure 4.3). Seven common misconceptions are critiqued in Pamphlet 16, entitled "The Best Food." They include the belief that the first days' breastmilk is of insufficient quantity and quality; that mothers who are malnourished produce poor milk; that some breasts produce little milk and quickly dry up; that when children cry, it is because they have not received enough milk; that if breasts are small, they cannot produce enough milk; that when mothers become angry, their milk becomes bad; that when a mother is ill, she should not breastfeed. The discussion shows why these beliefs are incorrect. The conclusion is that more mothers should give the breast so that when their children grow up, they will do the same with their children.

Somoza-style dictatorships and imperialism are frequently cited as examples of political and economic structures which contribute to ill health. In Pamphlet 7,

Popular Education 71

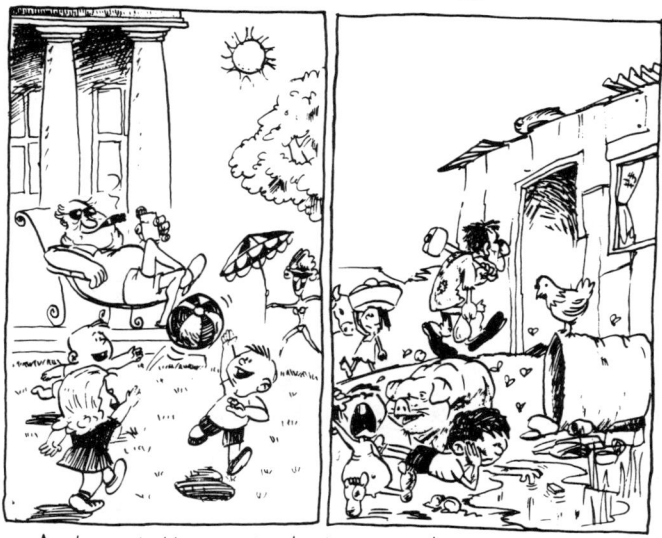

FIGURE 4.1: "Guide to read and study this pamphlet.
1. Read slowly. 2. When we have a question, we should answer it before continuing to read. 3. If we are in a group, each person should answer the question. At the end, try to formalize one answer on the basis of what each one said. 4. Continue reading and check to see if the answers which we gave are correct."

"Analyze the questions and discuss the questions: Which of these children are more apt to become ill from diarrhea? Why are the living conditions of these children different?"

72   The Nicaraguan Revolution in Health

"For this reason the Revolution is taking steps to eliminate exploitation and improve living conditions."

"We can see some of the changes already and what they have accomplished."

(signs:)

-National Literacy Campaign

-Popular Health Campaigns

-Oral Rehydration Units

-Cooperatives

-Agrarian Reform

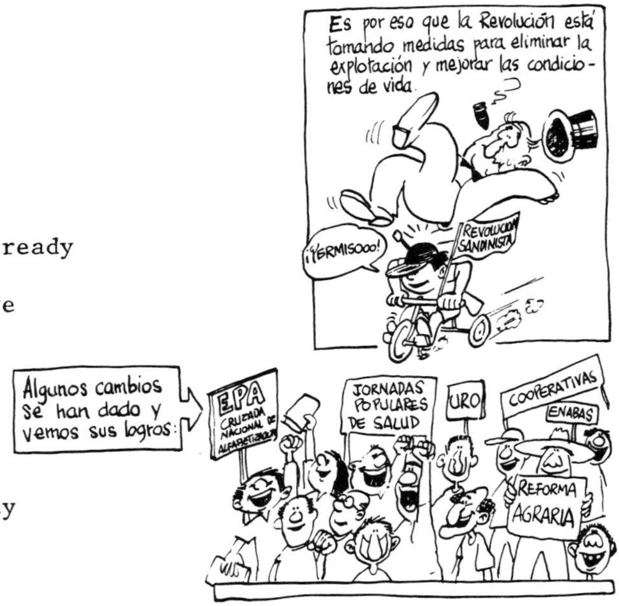

FIGURE 4.2

Popular Education 73

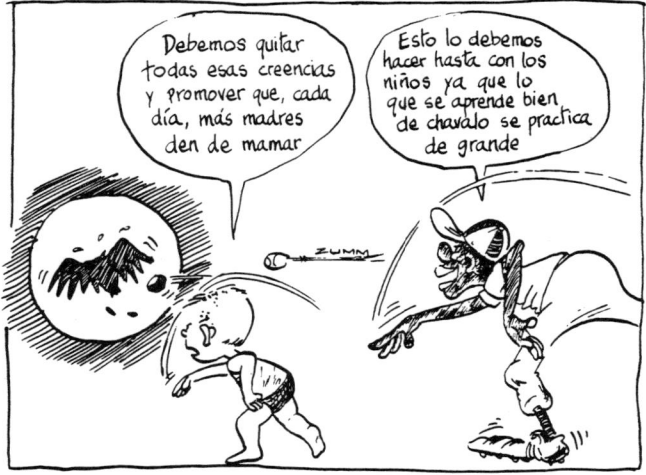

FIGURE 4.3: "We ought to rid ourselves of all these beliefs and see to it that every day more mothers breastfeed."
"We should do this with the youngsters so that what they learn to do well as children, they will practice as adults."

entitled "Water," the discussants recall that in the past monies for potable water systems were pocketed by the Somocistas (Figure 4.4).

Economic and geographical inaccessibility to health providers is another structural cause of illness. In Pamphlet 9, entitled "Life, Pain and Death of the Teeth," there is a discussion of why the teeth of Nicaraguans are on the average in such poor condition. The major cause is found in the characteristics of prerevolutionary dentistry in Nicaragua: poor training of dentists, the poor distribution of dentists in the country, and the fee-for-service and restorative focus of dentistry (Figure 4.5).

Protagonists in the pamphlets constantly model the dialogue which is to go on in the group during the thematic decoding and structural analysis. To mention only a few cases, dialogues occur between children and the Brigadista, between a baseball player and a child (Figure 4.3 above), and two boys and a crippled man who discuss polio (Figure 4.6). One boy, crippled from polio, explains to the healthy boy how the disease is transmitted. An older man in a wheelchair describes what anguish a polio victim causes among family members. The crippled boy cheers up his healthy friend and encourages him to receive the oral vaccine. The man lectures the two boys from his wheelchair on the seven steps to be taken to organize their neighborhood for the national polio vaccination campaign.

The antithesis of dialogue, the traditional talk by a professional, is satirized in Pamphlet 1. The protagonist, a comical, cross-eyed figure ("el chaquite"), is constantly interrupted by the members of the Popular Health Council. They freely offer their comments and observations.

Group summaries are frequently used to reinforce discussion points. Several times during the reading of a pamphlet the group will be advised to stop, and not continue until they have thoroughly discussed the question at hand. An example is found in a summary statement regarding rehydration (see Figure 4.7). Mothers are advised to expect that children will pass much of the oral rehydration (URO) that they receive. Nevertheless, more liquid will stay in the body than will be lost. Like a jar with a hole in it, the water level will be maintained as long as more water is added than is lost. If the child vomits, one should wait twenty minutes, give him air and repeat the URO in small doses. After three to six hours the child should be rehydrated.

Another principle of health education is that the materials must originate with and return to the popular

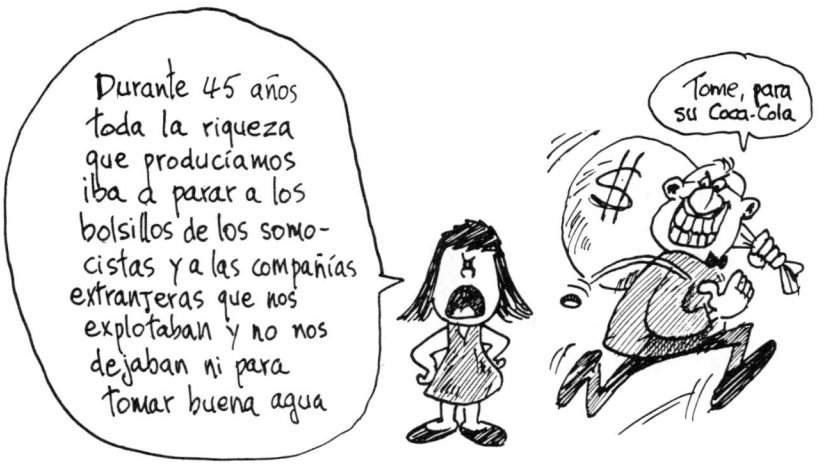

FIGURE 4.4: "For 45 years all the wealth we produced went into the pockets of the Somocistas and the foreign companies which exploited us and they did not leave enough even to drink good water."

"Take this for your coca-cola."

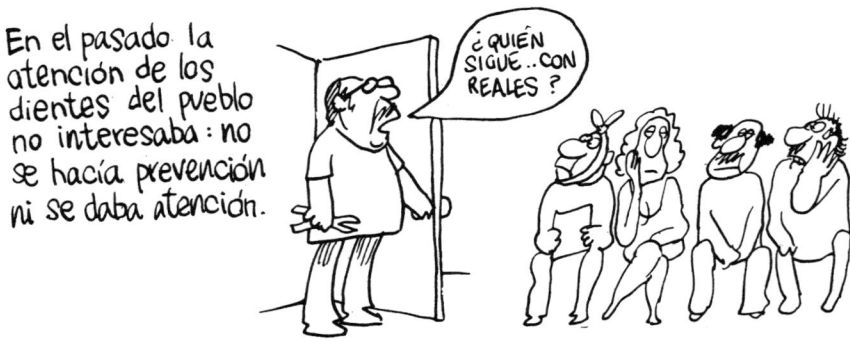

FIGURE 4.5: "In the past there was no interest in the dental care of the people: there was no prevention nor were dental services offered."

"Who's next...with money?"

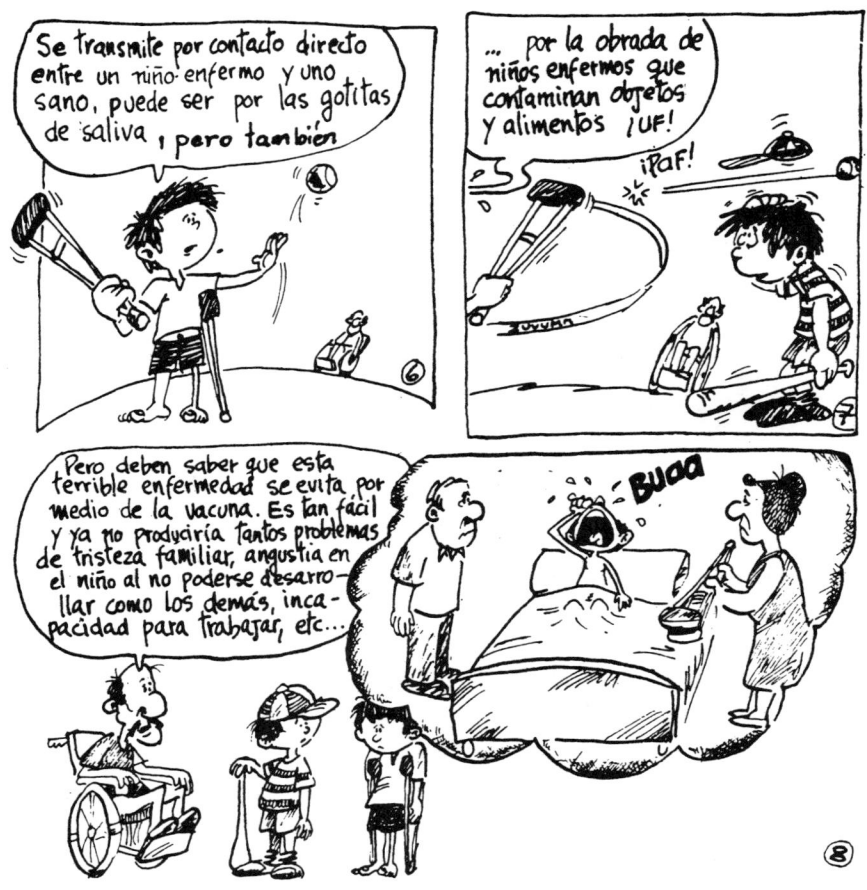

FIGURE 4.6: "Polio is transmitted by direct contact between a sick child and a healthy one be it by drops of saliva...or by the excrement of sick children which contaminates objects and foods. Uuf!"

"But you should know that this terrible illness is avoided by means of a vaccine. It is so easy and there will be no more family sadness, no more anxiety for the child who cannot develop like the rest, no more inability to work, etc...."

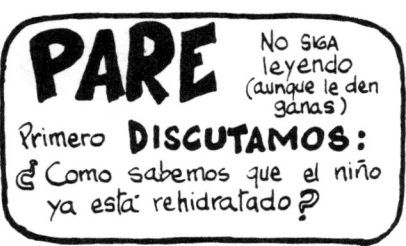
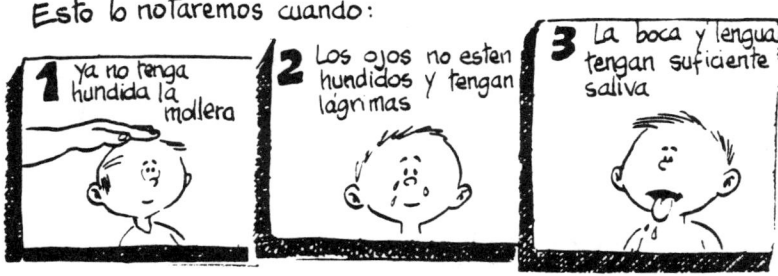

FIGURE 4.7: "Stop! Do not continue reading (although you may wish to). First, let's discuss: How do we know that a child is now rehydrated?"

"Generally, after 3 to 6 hours, the child will be rehydrated. We know this when: 1. The soft spot is no longer sunken. 2. The eyes are no longer sunken and they have tears. 3. The mouth and tongue have sufficient saliva..."[continued] classes. One of the assumptions of the decoding process is that the codes must be themselves culturally relevant to the participants. Not only must they speak to their experience, but they should also elicit a feeling that will energize the dialogue and eventually lead to an action that will transform the problem-posing reality.

The Pamphlets are replete with traditional cultural themes. Baseball sets the scene for several actors. Local foods and drinks appear. Somoza, a folk figure of all that is contrary to good health, is frequently ridiculed, as are critics of the health programs, such as opposition newspapers and some religious sects. Customs that endanger health, such as drunkenness and "wives tales" are addressed. Housing conditions, street vendors, and local animals are familiar images in the pamphlets. In addition to these traditional cultural images, the Revolution has brought new components to popular culture such as a redefinition of women's roles (Figure 4.8).

Another element added to popular cultural themes is the defense of the revolution by the Popular Militia. The analogy used to describe the interaction of antibodies and germs draws upon the experience of the popular militia in identifying and extracting the Somocista counter-revolutionaries as they infiltrate back into the country (Figure 4.9).

The military analogy extends to the antimalaria campaign which is seen as the "final offensive." Bacteria, the "enemies of food," are described in terms reminiscent of the "enemies of the revolution." In all of these cases the effort is to use a cultural idiom taken from the people so that their problem-posing and problem-solving can take place in that same idiom.

Finally, the educational materials should have popular organization and collective action as the central and unifying theme. Popular education is political education in the sense that the improvement of health depends in great part on the ability of the disadvantaged to become conscious of their power to transform their less human conditions into more human conditions. In this sense the materials should follow the logic of the learning process, i.e. from the known to the unknown, from the easily understood to the more difficult, from the near at hand to the more distant, from mere description to analysis, from observation to interpretation, and from unicausality to multicausality. This power to transform rests not only in the intellect, but also in the will. Hence, the educational materials must lead the people to political organization and action on behalf of

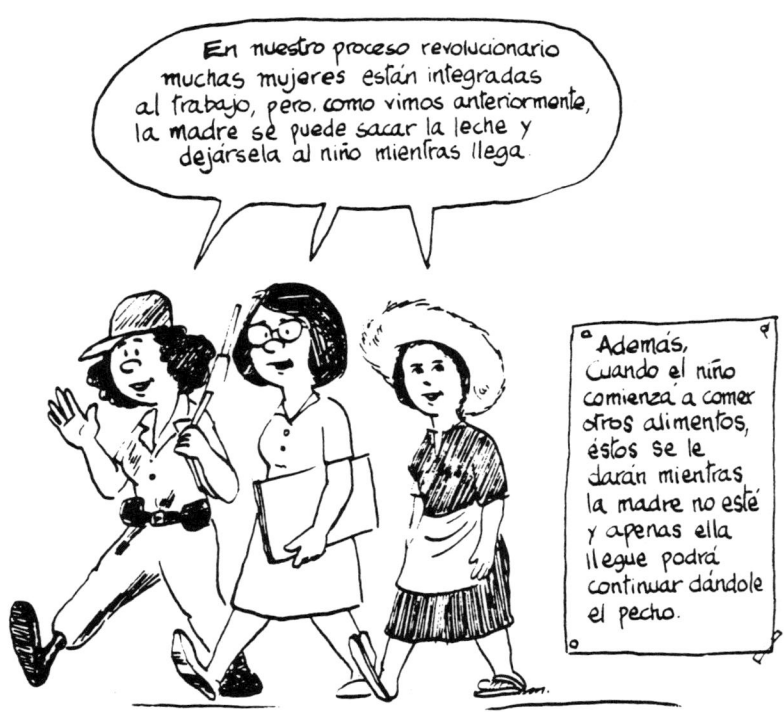

FIGURE 4.8: "In our revolutionary process many women are part of the work force, but, as we have seen above, a mother can remove some milk and leave it for the child until she gets home."

"Besides, when the child begins to eat other foods, these can be given while the mother is away. As soon as she arrives, she can continue to give the breast."

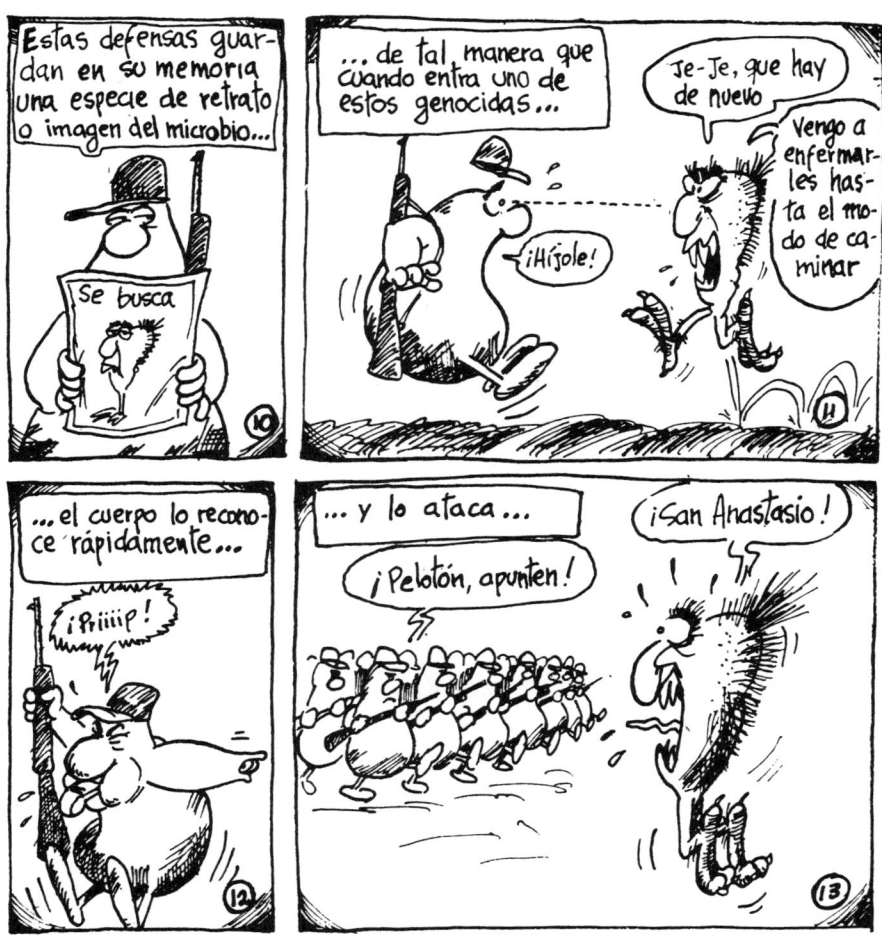

FIGURE 4.9: "These defenses maintain in their memory a kind of picture or image of the microbe..." "...such that when one of these killers..." "Hey. Hey, what's new...I've come to make you sick, even the way you walk." "...the body recognizes the microbe immediately..." "...and attacks it..." "The bald one... Take aim!" "Saint Anastasius!"

their own health.

The participation message of the Health Pamphlets and Documents is coded in a generative theme we may refer to as "social medicine." One of the principle characteristics of this theme is that the power of health rests ultimately not in the hands of physicians, but of the people themselves.

The pamphlet "What are the Popular Health Commissions," discusses the role of government and people in health before and after the revolution. The dialogue takes place between a young man and an elderly woman who asks what the Popular Health Commissions are all about. In return for a glass of tiste (a local corn drink), the young man concedes to her request. He asks her to describe how the Somoza government cared for health. She describes its hospital focus and the preferential treatment given to the National Guard. A third person remarks that the Guard bombed some hospitals during the war. She recalls how during the insurrection Radio Sandino advised people how to prevent epidemics. The Sandinists ("Los Muchachos") taught first aid to the people in the barrios. The young man remarks that since the revolution, government and people have come together in the Popular Health Councils to propose, discuss, and plan health programs. Health is no longer an act of charity, a gift from Santa Claus or a private service available only to those who can pay. Prevention does not depend on thousands of doctors, but on the organization of people who work together to create healthy living conditions (Figure 4.10).

Good health is a question of prevention, a task which depends for success on organization. Specific attention is given to personal activities which can prevent illness, such as care of food and water and breastfeeding. Even some curative medicine is in the power of the people, be it the treatment of dehydration due to diarrhea or first aid for minor emergencies. Groups are often asked, "What can we do to multiply this knowledge?" Prevention is a collective responsibility and the dissemination of health knowledge and action further guarantees the people's health.

The analysis of Popular Health education and activity in Nicaragua suggests several observations on the replicability of the experience in other developing countries. The first relates to the fundamental political nature of health education and activity. The decision of governments to organize and train large segments of the population for disease prevention and primary care is clearly a political one, not only to initiate the process, but to abide by the popular demands which will arise as a

Popular Education   83

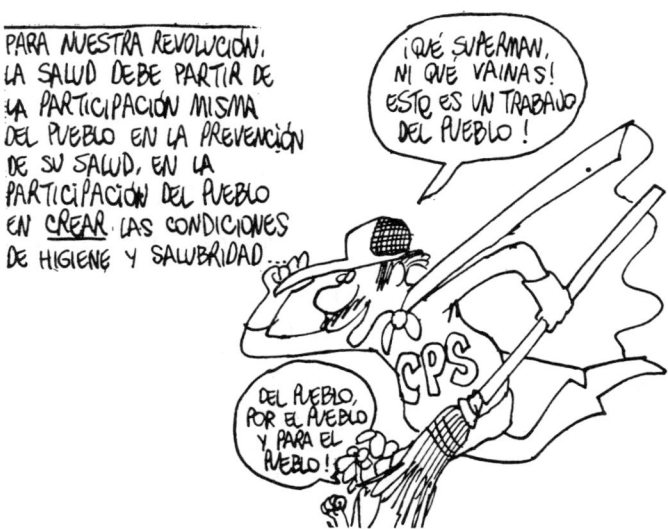

"For our revolution in
health must begin with
the participation of the
people in prevention, in
the participation of the
people in the creation
of health and well being
..."

"This is not the work
of a superman or the
like, but of the
people..."

"...Of the people,
by the people, and
for the people."

FIGURE 4.10

consequence. Once organized by government to address health issues, however, people may turn their popular organizations to other issues such as education, wages, and agrarian reform. Governments which organize people for health must be ready for the democratizing demands of those organizations in other sectors as well.

A second lesson of popular education in Nicaragua is that massive health organization and participation must have a special character in societies highly stratified into sectors of a very wealthy minority and a very poor majority. In such circumstances, popular health education must direct people to the reform of those social, economic, and political structures that stand between them and their health. For popular education to be political education, the poor and sick must ultimately take collective action on their own behalf.

A final observation relates to the relationship of popular health education to professional providers, and the institutional interests present in the health sector. In many developing countries primary health care has been "professionalized" and made dependent on elaborate medical referral systems. There is a growing awareness that the referral process of patients through clinics and hospitals may never get off the ground without effective local organization and participation in out-reach programs (England 1978; Donahue 1981). Local support depends upon nonprofessional involvement in preventive and some curative tasks. Yet, such active involvement may threaten the traditional control of medical providers and health professionals over the setting of health priorites in general and their institutional interests in particular. The case of Nicaragua suggests that even in a country where popular organizations and participation have brought vast improvements in the general health of the population, the issue of professional/popular control is still not settled.

NOTES

[1] One of the major actors in and commentators on the National Literacy Crusade is Oscar Jara, a Peruvian and student of Freire, who had extensive experience in popular education in Peru and Chile. Jara (1981) has summarized the experience of many in the National Literacy Crusade. Several of his observations on the preparation of teaching materials

were incorporated into efforts to design a program in popular education in health in 1980 and 1981. Since that time Jara has served as a consultant to the Division of Communication and Popular Education in Health (DECOPS) and the Center for Investigations and Studies of the Agrarian Reform (CIERA).

[2] It was at this time that the idea was conceived to compose illustrated health pamphlets that would be interesting and simply written so as to engage a population that had only recently become literate (MINSA 1980c:39). Several of the pamphlets were illustrated by the Chilean artist Miguel Marfan and Rius, a pseudonym for Eduardo del Rio. Rius, a Mexican caricaturist and editorial cartoonist, is the creator of the political and documentary cartoon-book. Among his works are Marx for Beginners (1976), Lenin for Beginners (1976), and Nicaragua for Beginners (1982).

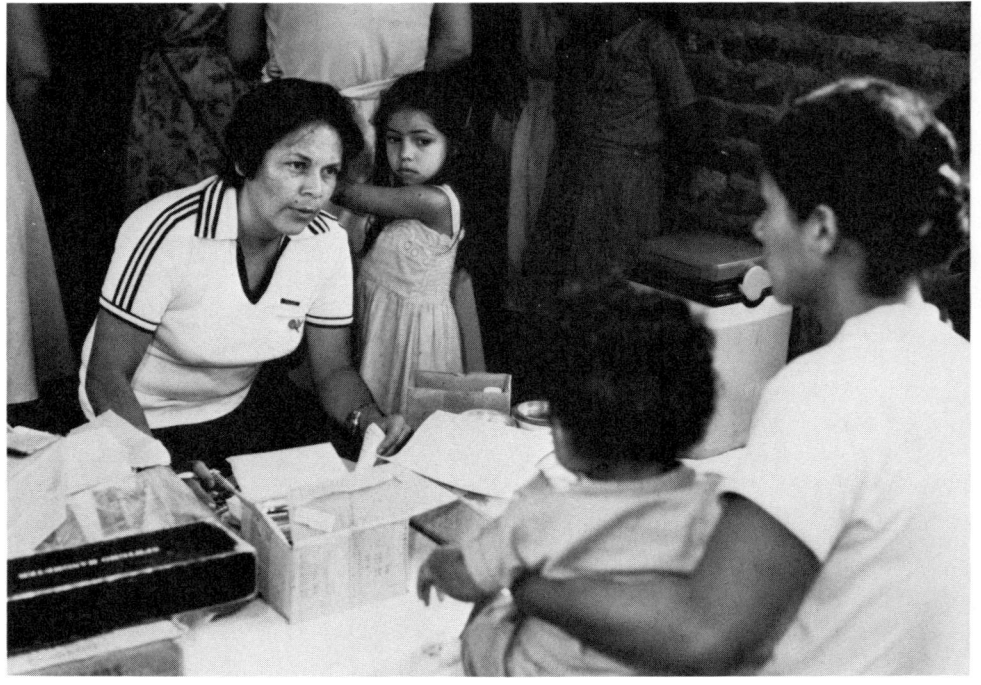
Auxiliary nurses make regular trips into the rural villages.

Chapter 5
COMPETING AGENDAS IN PRIMARY HEALTH CARE

RURAL AND URBAN HEALTH NEEDS

The success of the Popular Health Days drew world-wide attention to the role of the popular participation in primary health care in Nicaragua. As a result, UNICEF chose Nicaragua to be one of several countries in which to demonstate a model primary health care delivery system. In March 1981 the World Health Organization, the Pan American Health Organization, and UNICEF entered into a dialogue with the Ministries of Health and Planning on primary health care strategies for Nicaragua (MIPLAN/MINSA 1981:7, MINSA n.d.). The discussions led to the presentation in April 1982 of the Comprehensive Plan for Assistance to Health Areas (PIAAS) by the Division of Primary Care (MINSA 1982b).

Two different points of view on primary health care had to be reconciled in the design and implementation of the national program. A major point of contention was the institutional focus of some medical professionals who envisioned the primary care worker (Brigadista) to be primarily an extension of the medical staff of the Area Health Clinic. (1) In contrast, the Division of Education and Popular Communication in Health (DECOPS) trained Health Workers to take their knowledge and multiply it through the training of yet other Health Workers. DECOPS stressed the

88 The Nicaraguan Revolution in Health

importance of training primary care workers to provide a range of services. In largely rural Nicaragua, direct care seemed a more realistic strategy than reliance on an urban model of medical referral (England 1978, Donahue 1981). The DECOPS model of primary care delivery drew upon the experience of the Popular Health Days in which prevention and health programs at the community level were given more prominence than the referral of patients to health facilities. The differences between the two approaches reflect two different models of primary care delivery. The one emphasizes medical control and supervision to insure quality care within a clinical setting. The other focuses more upon the dissemination of health knowledge and both preventive and curative health services in nonclinical settings. Before we look more closely at the two models, we need to understand the different experiences in grass roots organization out of which they were born.

BACKGROUND TO DIFFERING MODELS

The intensity of the National Guard's repressive tactics was greater on the Pacific than on the Atlantic coast. As a result, Nicaraguans on the Pacific coast developed a more extensive grass roots political and military organization than those who lived on the Atlantic coast. After the insurrection, political activity in the popular organizations was more widespread and easily mobilized for health delivery on the Pacific coast than along the Atlantic. In the health sector an institutional primary care plan resonated with the grass roots political organization, vertical integration, and patterns of participation found on the Pacific side of the country. By contrast, an alternative experience and model of health activity was needed among the peoples living on the Atlantic coast.

The Atlantic coast represents one half of the national territory, but less than one tenth of the total population. An English-speaking creole and indigenous population of Miskitu, Sumu, and Rama peoples live in dispersed settlements and family households along the many rivers that flow to the Atlantic. There are several major urban settlements, but the vast majority of the population lives in isolated rural areas. The relative isolation of the peoples of the Atlantic coast also helps explain why under Somoza they received few services of any kind (Helms 1982:72, 91). Several Protestant churches, notably the

Moravians, provided the only educational and health services available.

One of the first organizing experiences after the revolution was the literacy campaign. The only effective way to reach the dispersed population on the Atlantic coast was through a network of local literacy workers. The strategy of networking was carried over and further refined in the Popular Health Days (Ellsberg 1983). The health workers in the Special Zone of South Zelaya on the Atlantic Coast were not able to designate specific days for the health campaigns. Longer periods of time were needed. The health brigadistas spread throughout the country and along the rivers, trained yet other brigadistas and organized the various campaigns. Fewer Popular Organizations existed on the Atlantic coast. Consequently, the health workers themselves were often responsible for the initial organization of the communities into Popular Health Councils (Ellsberg 1982). Thus health services and not political consciousness or mass organizations became the principal vehicle for popular organization along the Atlantic Coast.

Another difference between the two primary health care experiences involved the relationship of primary care workers to health care professionals. The national health education program for the Health Days envisioned a process whereby health educators would be quickly trained throughout the country. Some 120 health educators were assigned to each Region. They provided extended training to volunteer personnel, referred to as "multipliers," whose task it would be to train the brigadistas at the local level. (2) The effect was to quickly disseminate information and training downward and outward from health educator, to multiplier, to brigadista. The program operated throughout the nation prior to each Popular Health Work Day and then ceased. In South Zelaya, however, the popular health education and service delivery program became a permanent feature of that Primary Health Care Program. During 1981, 196 health brigadistas from 135 communities were organized into a pyramidal structure for training and delivery purposes. At the base were the local Popular Health Councils which were then organized into Health Brigades of eight to ten brigadistas and brought together into periodic Area Assemblies and Regional Congresses (Ellsberg 1982). The health brigadista collaborated at each level with Ministry personnel, but the brigadista, and not the health professional, was the focal point of the entire primary health care effort.

Brigadistas in the health clinics in the western half of the country were more often representatives of the clinic and its staff. By contrast, health brigadistas in South Zelaya were far from health facilities and medical staff. Health educators from the Ministry encouraged them to disseminate health education and to deliver primary care to as many people as possible. The result has been the growth of an extensive network of Health Brigadistas throughout the Atlantic coastal area, many of whom were themselves trained not by Ministry personnel but by other Brigadistas.

Proponents of the South Zelaya primary care model within the Ministry of Health in Managua criticized the institutional approach on five counts. (3) First, they argued that the initial draft of the PIAAS manual (MINSA 1982b) revealed an institutional approach that emphasized brigadista training from a biomedical perspective; in contrast, the South Zelaya model recommended training that would focus upon the social and environmental dimensions of illness and disease. Second, the manual placed greater emphasis on administrative matters and professional control than on continuing popular education. Third, the institutional approach seemed less concerned with a conscious and critical political education which could critize, if necessary, the health professional and the Ministry itself. Fourth, there was concern that the Health Brigadistas and midwives would be used only until there were sufficient health professionals. Finally, the dichotomy between primary health care, health education and training seemed to be too rigid. According to one International Health Advisor, the Division of Primary Health Care should be more than just another office within the Ministry of Health; it should be the fundamental strategy of the entire health sector in Nicaragua. As such, primary health care would reach beyond the clinics into other institutional settings such as schools, factories, farms, and neighborhoods.

RESOLUTION OF THE CONFLICT

Discussions continued within the Ministry in search for a more broadly defined primary care strategy. As a result, there emerged an approach to primary health care and health brigadista training that altered the conditions of professional dominance inherent in the original PIAAS Area Clinic structure. The protagonist for the more popular strategy has been the Division of Education and Popular Communication in Health. In July 1983 DECOPS was able to present to the Ministry and the Popular Health Councils their proposed "Strategy for Popular Training in Primary

Health Care in Nicaragua" (DECOPS/MINSA 1983). As will be discussed below, primary health care programs must now compete with demands for emergency and acute care of those affected by increasing contra hostilities. Yet, the DECOPS plan serves as the basis for a comprehensive primary care approach, once Nicaragua is allowed to return to its peacetime reform programs.

The popular health model differs from the institutional approach in five important respects:

I. Cultural authority is shifted from the professional-medical model to a social and popular health model. According to the model proposed by the Division of Popular Education, responsibility for the variety of primary health care tasks is to reside in the community and the popular organizations and not in the area clinic staff and programs. The tasks for which the community and its Health Brigadista are principally responsible include:

1. Health education
2. Nutrition care and supplemental food distribution
3. Potable water and environmental sanitation
4. Mother and child care
5. Immunization
6. Prevention and control of communicable diseases
7. Simple curative procedures
8. Basic medicines

II. Organizational realignments move the health delivery system beyond the area clinic. The popular model envisions that the four principle actors in primary health care will coordinate and integrate their efforts. They are governmental sectors other than the Ministry of Health, the Popular Health Councils, the Clinic Team and the health brigadistas. The organizational locus of coordination is the Popular Health Council. Its responsibilities include coordination of efforts among local institutions, the selection and training of health brigadistas, community organization and evaluation of primary care tasks (DECOPS/MINSA 1983). For its part, the Clinic Team is repsonsible for training and advising the Health Councils. They also provide technical training, support and supervision to the health brigadistas. The health educator, a member of the Clinic Team, has principal responsibility for coordination of efforts of the medical professionals, the Health Council, and the brigadista.

III. An expanded role and coverage is given to the

health brigadista. The vertical and subordinate role of the health brigadista in the original PIAAS program is changed in several ways. In the first place, the Primary Care Health Brigadista is recognized as being the principal point of contact between the community and the National Unified Health System (SNUS). In recognition of that fact, the role of the Primary Care Brigadista is broadened as regards both tasks and coverage. Tasks include education, prevention, health care delivery, and administration. Accordingly, the types of Primary Care Brigadista have been expanded to include multiple specialities such as sanitation, maternal-child care, school health, occupational health, and midwifery, as well as the Clinic Area Brigadista envisioned by the PIAAS program.

IV. The relationship of physician-nurse-brigadista in the areas of supervision and evaluation is redefined. Coverage is broadened also so as to provide a total of 41,400 Primary Care Brigadistas (BAPs) within several speciality areas. Training would cover four levels and be aimed at service to six target groups. All BAPS would receive Level I training in environmental sanitation. Of those, 12,500 would carry out those tasks in a permanent fashion as Sanitation Brigadistas (BS). The remaining 28,900 will receive Level II training in community health. Of those, 10,000 will carry out the tasks of Communal Brigadista (BC) within the neighborhood Sandinista Defense Committee. The BC is the coordinator of the activities of the other BAPS and the local health council. Level III training is given to the remaining 18,900 BAPS. Of these, 2000 will offer care to mothers and children as Mother-Child Brigadistas (BM-I). The rest will receive Level IV training to become Health Brigadistas for other target groups: School Brigadistas (BES-6800), Work Brigadistas (BOS-3500), Brigadistas for Area Health Clinics (BPIAAS-3600), and Midwives (PEA-3000).

V. The relationship of health professionals to health brigadistas is also redefined. In the institutional hierarchy of physician-nurse-brigadista, supervision implies the control of subordinates by superiors. The superior acts as a judge in evaluating the performance of subordinates measured against goals and objectives. As subordinate health workers account for their performance in this authoritarian management scheme, they may well acquiesce to professional authority in nonmedical as well as medical matters. As sometimes happens, the superior technical knowledge of the health professional may be converted into broader cultural authority over matters other than health, such as political power and social status. In the popular health model supervision and evaluation are to feature the sharing of information among health personnel, team effort and problem solving. Professional privilege, which impedes popular participation and community control, is to be eschewed.

In summary, the popular model is more compatible with the health needs of the largely rural population of Nicaragua. The institutional model is an example of urban bias in rural primary health care delivery. A decentralized health care program that utilizes trained primary care workers can reach more prople with a greater variety of services than urban-based clinical care alone.

PROBLEMS THAT REMAIN

In July of 1984 a reorganization of the Ministry was underway. A Ministry official explained that the objective was to provide for more efficiency in reporting within each Region. At the time, some nine offices, each with its own Director, reported to the Regional Health Director. The reorganization envisioned only four offices: Primary Care, Preventive Medicine, Medical Instruction ("Docencia") and Finance. The other five would report to the Regional Health Director through one of the those four offices. The Sub-Division of Education and Popular Education in Health (SECOPS) would no longer report directly to the Regional Health Director, but indirectly through the Director of the Office of Medical Instruction. The change may improve the coordination of activities between health educators and medical professionals within the Ministy. On the other hand, the change may spell a loss of autonomy for health educators. Their access to the Regional Health Director will now be through the office whose primary responsibility is for medical school education.

Current political and military conditions in Central America are already adversely affecting the popular health care model. The United States economic boycott of Nicaragua has contributed to shortages of medical supplies, pharmaceuticals and paper used in popular education and normal day-to-day administrative operations. The undeclared war of the Unites States against Nicaragua had created some 120,600 internal refugees by May 1984 (INSSBI 1984:7) and absorbed $66 million dollars in relief and relocation costs

(INSSBI 1984:9). By mid-1984 the damages inflicted upon the health infrastructure by the contras amounted to $1 million dollars (INSSBI: 1984:12). Twenty health centers had been closed in the Special Zone of North Zelaya and in Region I (Esteli) near the Honduran border (INSSBI 1984: 12-13). At the same time, increased contra activity in the country has created a demand for emergency and surgical care (Garfield 1985:123).

Correspondingly, priorities for brigadista training have changed. By July 1984, some 20,000 Primary Care Brigadistas had been trained in first aid, primarily to assist war casualities. The training of mother-child Brigadistas had lagged. Training of School and Work Brigadistas had yet to begin in earnest. Meanwhile, in some areas of the country, increased civilian and military casualities contributed, in part, to the allocation of more resources to secondary than to primary care. In Region II (Leon-Chinandega) fully 60 percent of the 1983 regional budget went to an acute care hospital (MINSA/Region II 1984).

On the other hand, the popular health model is proving its vitality even in the face of these difficult circumstances. The labor intensive nature of the primary care program allowed Region II to surpass its goal of prenatal encounters (MINSA/Region II 1984). The Sub-Division of Education and Popular Communication in Health reported that in 1983, 89.6 percent and 93 percent of children were vaccinated against polio in two campaigns and 87 percent in an anti-measles vaccination program (SECOPS/Region II 1984).

A health educator reported that a brigadista from Cinco Pinos near the border with Honduras was going house to house as part of his vaccination schedule. Several families in one isolated hamlet were especially grateful, remarking that it was the first time that they had ever been visited by a health worker. The brigadista then learned that he had strayed into Honduras.

The popular model is proving viable even in the face of hostilities within the Central American region. In July 1984 there was an outbreak of polio in Honduras. The Honduran Ministry of Health accepted an initial 50,000 doses of oral vaccine from the Nicaraguan Ministry of Health with another 500,000 to follow. The Hondurans welcomed, as consultants, the Nicaraguan Chief Epidemiologist and the National Director of DECOPS (Nuevo Diario June 30, 1984).

SUMMARY

Several conclusions can be drawn from the discussion. The first concerns the relevance of the conflict between models of primary care delivery to the study of change within health systems. The ascendancy of the Division of Popular Education model of primary care and the role of the Popular Health Councils suggest that the Nicaraguan health system is moving toward a model of primary health care that is decentralized and orientated to local needs, especially in the rural areas. Yet, within the Ministry itself there are interests which could direct the health care system more to urban and professional demands. The training of large numbers of Nicaraguan physicians (5) and the presence of many physicians in Nicaragua from other countries suggests that a medical professionalism might eventually dominate health planning and delivery within the national health system (Bossert 1984, 1985).

Second, it should come as no surprise that the final version of the Comprehensive Plan for Assistance to Health Areas (PIAAS) was the result of competition between two models of primary health care training and delivery in Nicaragua. Issues related to professionalism in primary health care are found in many developing countries, including China (Rosenthal and Greiner 1982:330-341). The Nicaraguan case may be unique in that there exists an institutionalized forum, the Popular Health Councils, in which the debate can be carried out. Within the public health bureaucracy itself the two models have their respective constituencies. The Division of Popular Communication and Education in Health exercises an advocacy role for a primary care model which places more emphasis upon the social and political dimensions of health and illness. Some medical professionals tend to promote a primary health care model which stresses access to clinical medicine and quality assurance. The conflict could produce a new synthesis in which clinical practice would be reconciled with popular participation, health education, and the widespread distribution of trained health workers in schools, factories, farms and neighborhoods.

The Government of National Reconstruction has not remained neutral in the struggle to create a participatory health delivery system. The 1981 appointment of Lea Guido, a woman and social scientist, to the post of Minister of Health signaled that the Ministry was to take a new direction. As a Cuban health advisor in Managua remarked, "More than twenty years have passed since our revolution, but we have yet to have a Minister of Health who is not a physician".

In May 1985 Commandante Dora Maria Tellez, herself a one-time medical student, replaced Ms. Guido as Minister of Health. The change was presented as a lateral one in which Guido and Tellez would simply exchange jobs, with Guido becoming overseer of the Ministry of Health for the Sandinista Party, a role that Tellez had held for several years. Yet, the change could be viewed within the context of the continuing pull between professional and popular agendas within the Ministry.

Among the issues that seem to underlie the change in Ministers was a perceived decline in morale among the members of the professional medical community. For instance, there was a small, but constant, exit of physicians from the country, due, in part, to personal and professional hardships. Physicians had been negotiating with the Sandinista leadership for preferential treatment in the purchase of vehicles and allocation of gasoline as well as educational and housing benefits for their families. For their part, the Sandinista leadership seemed to be concerned with bureaucratic inefficiencies and the need to correct previous policies of hospital expansion (Ortega 1985).

The change in Ministers may have been a signal to the professional community that certain concessions would be made to the physicians, but that everyone should expect a tightening up of the administrative bureauracy, more emphasis on outreach and rural service, and a reaffirmation of the popular agenda in health care.

The strides made in health care since 1979 are abundant evidence of the political will to improve the health and well-being of the Nicaraguan people. Yet, the ultimate success of the revolution in health will depend on how the actors are able to confront the internal pressures to professionalize the process and the external pressures to destabilize it.

NOTES

[1] Scholl (1985) cites an interview with the Director of the Division of Primary Care which represents this point of view.

[2] See Table 3.1 in Chapter 3 for the summary statistics of personnel trained during 1981.

[3] The following obervations represent those of the author, based upon interviews with Ministry personnel, representatives of the Popular Organizations and with international health personnel, some of whom worked within the Ministry and others who worked for International Health Agencies.

[4] A second medical school has been established in Managua. Both schools have increased enrollments of entering medical students to 500.

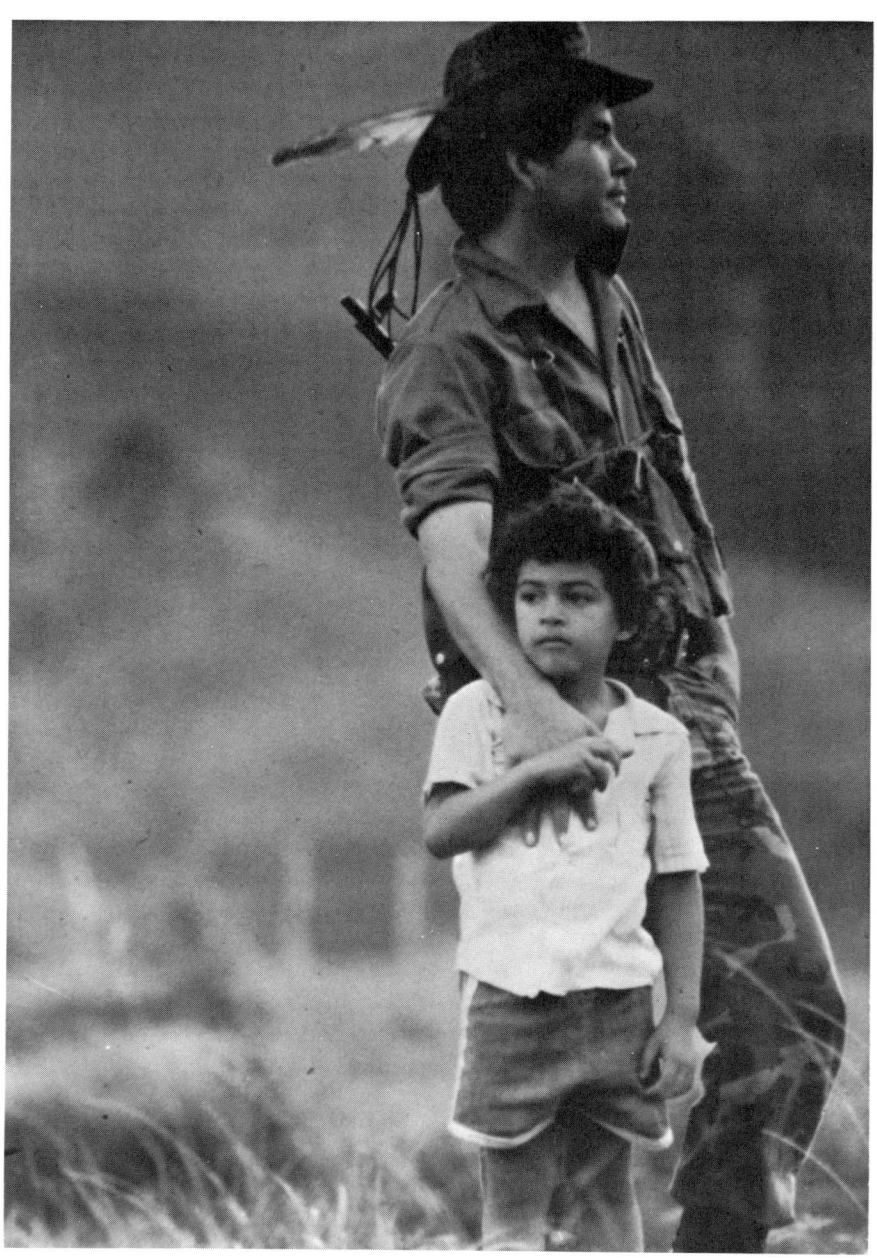
A father and son stand watch at Jalapa on the border with Honduras from where *contras* launch attacks aimed at clinics and health personnel.

Chapter 6
CONCLUSION: LESSONS FOR THE FUTURE

The experiences of the Popular Health Days, the Popular Health Councils, and brigadista training each reveal a host of popular agendas, including interest group organizations, paramedical training, professional accountability and popular health education and practice. The competition between professional and populist agendas is negotiated in each of the areas. Indeed, an analysis of strategies of popular participation suggest that the populist agendas must continually compete with professional efforts to redirect them to institutionalist goals such as the construction of urban hospitals. That this competition can take place in public fora such as the Popular Health Councils at various levels is itself a measure of the success of the Sandinista revolution in decentralizing the decision-making process. The outcome for the health system as a whole is not yet discernable for both internal and external reasons.

The Nicaraguan case demonstrates the need to study the process of change, rather than to rely solely on such health system descriptions as "nationalized," "socialized," or "in transition." An analysis of the process of change within Nicaragua suggests that the revolution in health, even in an optimal "decentralized-concerted" political environment (Elling 1980:106-107), is being negotiated. If one were to analyze the Nicaraguan health system from a structural point of view alone, one might conclude with Bossert (1984:73-74) that Nicaragua has not achieved the restructuring necessary to reduce future health care problems and redirect resources away from urban hospital health care. An analysis of the process of change reveals that the restructuring is still underway as different interest groups attempt to influence the direction of change.

The Nicaraguan case suggests that physicians are not being "deprofessionalized," but have been quite able to exercise their influence within the nationalized health system. They are being made more accountable through formal administrative and bureaucratic mechanisms, such as the Popular Health Councils (Freidson 1970:160). The new structures of citizen participation may make professionals more sensitive to he national goals of health care and the concrete means of implementing them at the local level. It remains to be seen what the long-range effects of community representation will have on the quality of care within the health system (Freidson 1970:212).

Elling notes that a health system, like the political economy in which it is embedded, is dynamic, and changes in accordance with internal pressures and the society's place within the world system (1980:107). Nicaragua's domestic revolution in health is no less immune from outside pressures that other dimensions of the national reform.

The undeclared war of the United States against Nicaragua, and its support of the contras, bears directly on the health of the Nicaraguan people. Health and education workers are special targets for contra assassinations (Siegel 1985:45). Civilian deaths due to contra activity number over 1,000 (Garfield and Taboada 1984:1143). Garfield (1985:127) estimates that war fatalities in Nicaragua among civilians and combatants has reached 10.0 per 10,000 and that more people are dying from the war than died from poliomyelitis, tetanus or measles before the revolution.

On the other hand, the popular health model is proving its vitality on an individual and group level even in the face of these difficult circumstances. Mobile health teams have been organized to work the villages normally serviced by the health posts closed down by the contras. Garfield and Taboada report that immunization coverage was higher in a war zone than in neighboring areas (1984:1143). It is ironic that after five years of reforms in the health sector, strategies first developed during the insurrection are proving to be once again viable alternatives to a beleaguered people.

There can be little doubt that the continued increase in military activities will reverse the achievements in health

CONCLUSION: LESSONS FOR THE FUTURE

of the last five years. There will be fewer resources for the health needs of the rural peoples as more national resources are allocated to defense, brigadistas are recruited into the armed services, and health facilities must of necessity treat the victims of war. Considering the health of Nicaraguans, the effect of the revolution has been a dramatic success, but one that is increasingly prone to reversal the longer the counterrevolution is waged.

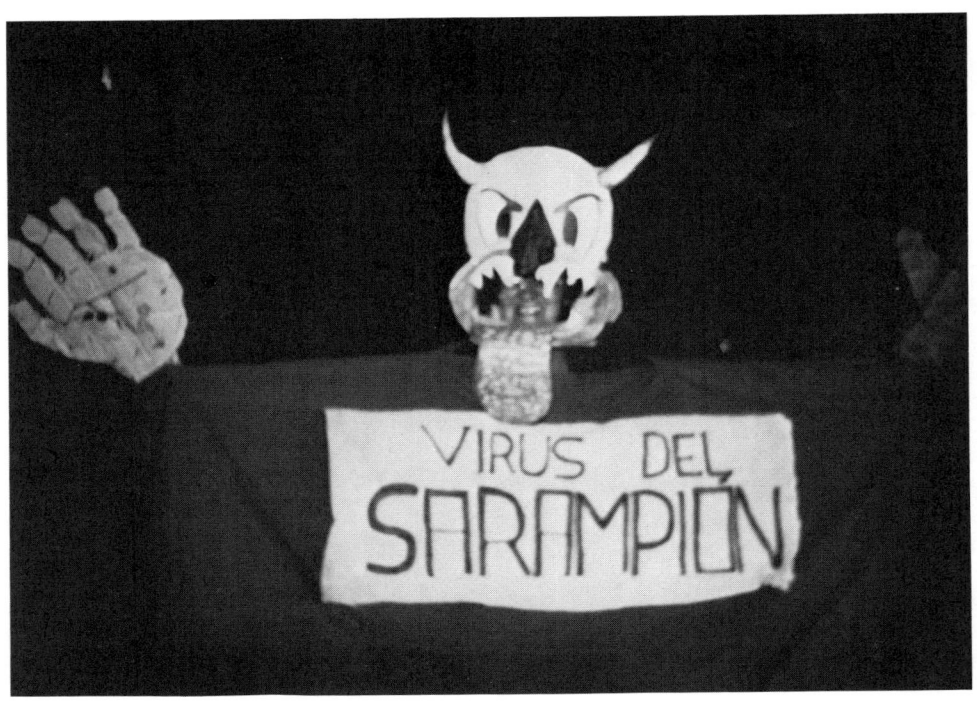
Maryknoll Sister Pat Edmisto plays the part of the measles virus during a popular health education drama.

Appendix A
HEALTH EDUCATION PAMPHLETS

Pamphlet 1 <u>Jornadas</u> <u>Populares</u> <u>de</u> <u>Salud</u>: <u>Que</u> <u>Son</u>...? (Popular Health Campaigns: What are They...?). 16 pages.

The pamphlet opens with two men chasing a fly ball. After a collision, they discuss their lack of coordination and discuss how health care, like baseball, is not learned from behind a desk, no matter how many the maps and statistics. Rather, it is the people who understand their health needs. They may not know what to do to meet them. The Popular Health Councils are described as the forums in which people can discuss and plan actions to solve their health needs. Class differentials in health status are addressed as well as class opposition to popular health activities.

104 The Nicaraguan Revolution in Health

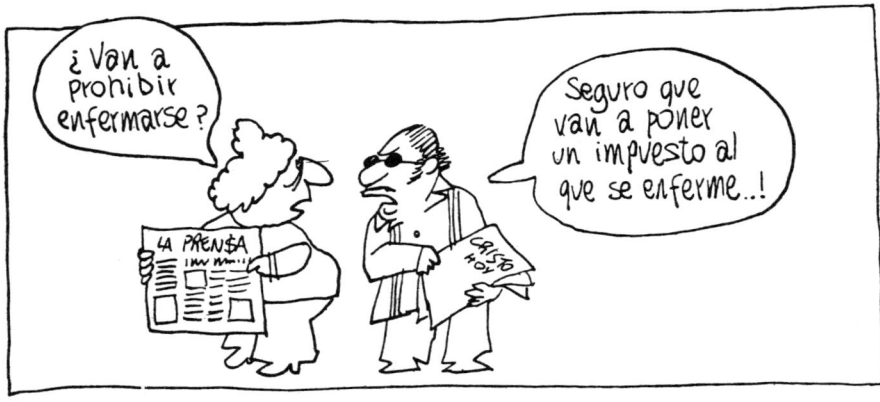

"Will they prohibit getting sick?"
"I think they're going to put a tax on the sick."

The second part of the pamphlet discusses at length the Popular Health Campaigns. The format is that of a read statement delivered to a meeting of a neighborhood Popular Health Council. The main protagonist is a comical figure called "Chibirizco el Bizco"(cross-eyed). At various points in the lecture, participants in the Council interrupt to offer comments or ask questions. Two themes are presented: the one suggests that only physicians can provide health care; the other argues that people, once organized, can educate others to care for their health.

Health Education Pamphlets 105

The discussion next turns to various mechanisms used in popular health organization and education. The first is the "multiplier" strategy in which 10 National Health educators train 12 Departmental counterparts. These in turn train 10 County-level Educators each for a total of 1200. Those train 20 "Health Brigadistas" each or 24,000 in all. The latter spread throughout their neighborhoods and rural villages with the message that "to produce health is to produce healthy living conditions." The three basic components of "health production" are cleanliness, vaccinations and proper diet. These become the three agendas of five Popular Health Campaigns to be carried out in 1981: the Anti-polio Vaccination, National Campaign of Environmental and Personal Hygiene, Anti-rabies Vaccination, Anti-malaria Campaign and the DPT Vaccination Campaign.

The final section describes how the Campaigns will be carried out with the use of mass communications, the popular organizations, the organization by the Health Brigadistas of local neighborhoods and villages into "columns" and "squadrons" and the coordinated efforts of the Ministry of Health and other governmental bodies.

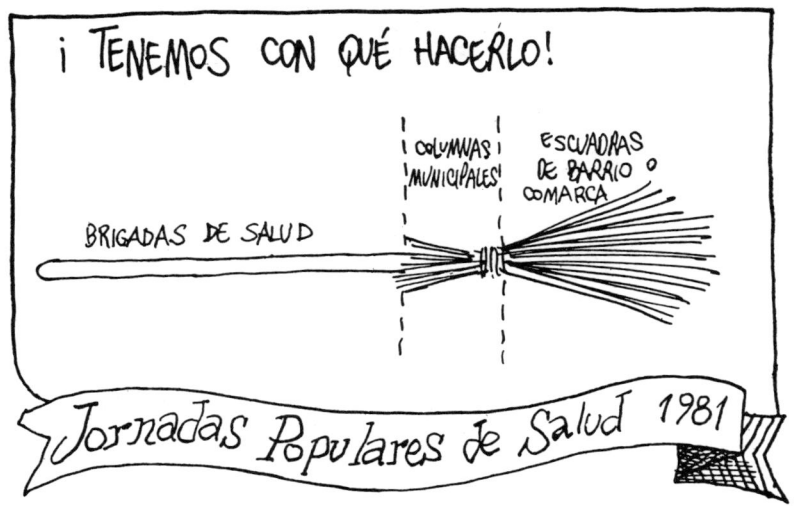

"We have what it takes!"
"Health Brigadistas...County Columns...Neighborhood Squadrons."
"Popular Health Days 1981"

106 The Nicaraguan Revolution in Health

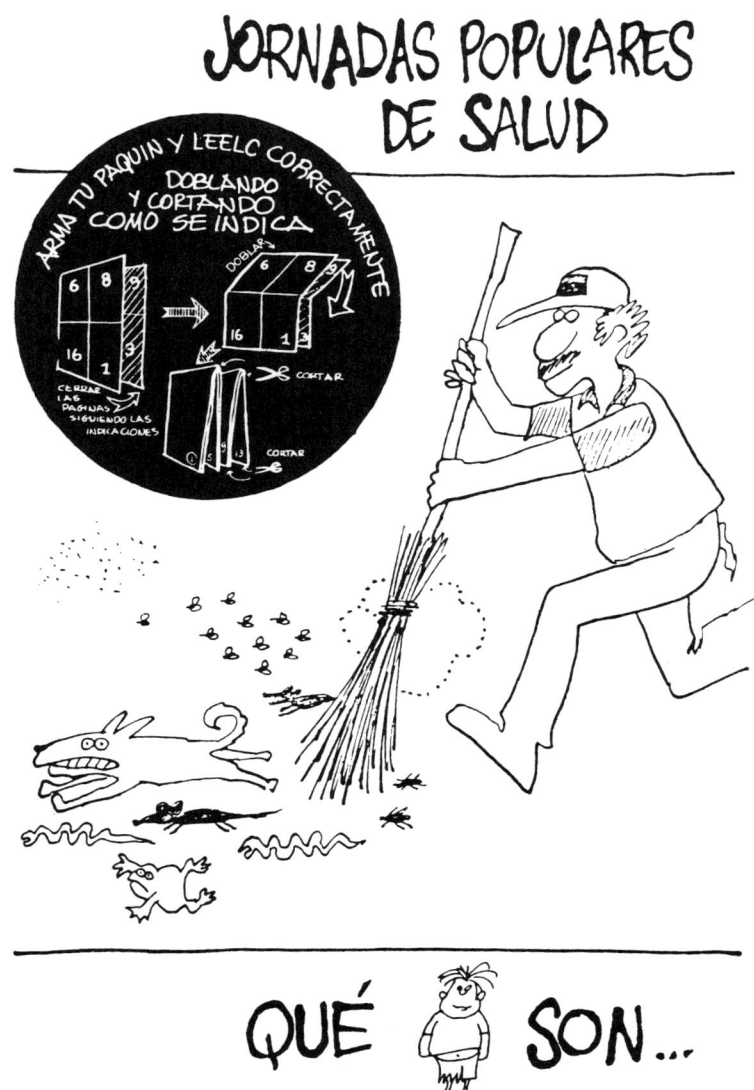

"Popular Health Days...What Are They?"

"Put together your pamphlet and read it correctly, folding and cutting it as indicated. Close the pages following the instructions, fold and cut."

Pamphlet 2. <u>Que</u> <u>Son</u> <u>Las</u> <u>Comisiones</u> <u>Populares</u> <u>de</u> <u>Salud</u>? (What are the Popular Health Commissions?). 4 pages.

This pamphlet discusses the role of government and people in health before and after the revolution. The dialogue takes place between a young man and an elderly woman who asks what the Popular Health Commissions are all about. In return for a glass of "tiste" (a local corn drink), the young man concedes to her request. He asks her to describe how the Somoza government cared for health. She describes its hospital focus and the preferential treatment given to the National Guard. A third person remarks that the Guard bombed some hospitals during the war. She recalls how during the insurrection Radio Sandino advised people how to prevent epidemics. The Sandinists ("Los Muchachos") taught first aid to the people in the barrios. The young man remarks that since the revolution, government and people have come together in the Popular Health Councils to propose, discuss and plan health programs. Health is no longer an act of charity, a gift from Santa Claus or a private service available only to those who can pay. Prevention does not depend on thousands of doctors, but on the organization of people who work together to create healthy living conditions.

108   The Nicaraguan Revolution in Health

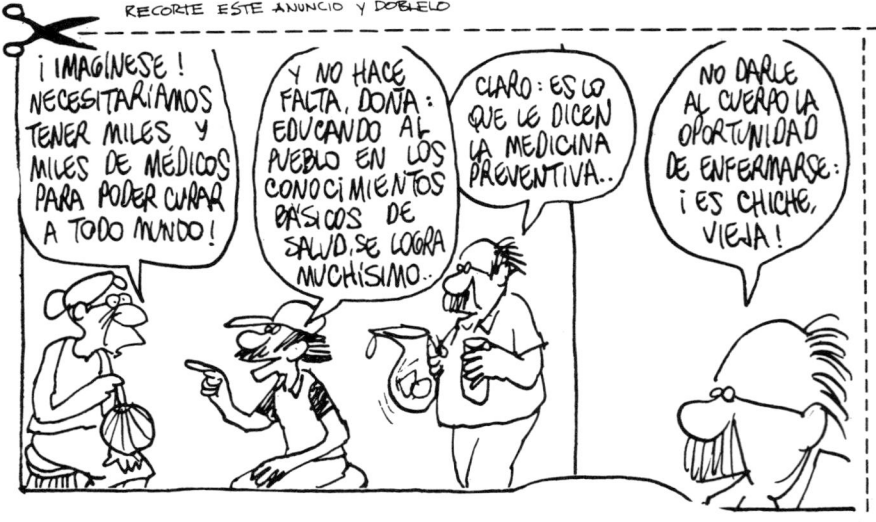

"Imagine! We would need to have thousands and thousands of doctors to be able to cure everyone." "And isn't it true, M'am, that educating people in basic health **principles**, one can accomplish much..." "You bet! This is what they call preventive medicine..." "Don't give the body an opportunity to become ill. That's the idea, madam."

Popular Health Pamphlets 109

Pamphlet 3 <u>Las Vacunas</u> (Vaccines). 4 pages.

This short description of vaccines includes an explanation of germ theory, how vaccines provide the individual with antibodies, why booster shots are necessary and against which illnesses vaccines protect both humans and animals. The analogy used to describe the interaction of antibodies and germs draws upon the experience of the popular militia in identifying and extracting the Somocista counter-revolutionaries as they infiltrate back into the country.

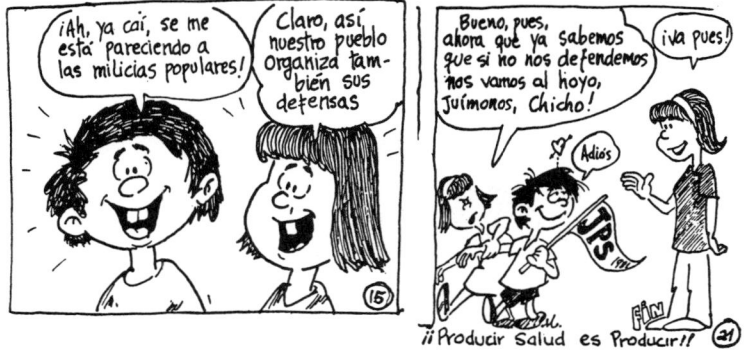

"Now I get it, they are like the popular militia."
"Sure. In this way people who are once organized have their own defense."

"OK. Now we know that if we don't defend ourselves, we'll end up in the grave. Let's get moving."

"Goodby." "See you." "To Produce Health is to Produce."

Pamphlet 4   La Polio (Polio). 8 pages.

   The discussion of the causes, effects, and prevention of polio are addressed to two audiences. The first is that of parents. The second is that of the local-level organizers of the "health posts" in which the vaccine will be administered. The format is a discussion between two young boys on a baseball playing field. The one, crippled from polio, explains to the healthy boy how the disease is transmitted. An older man in a wheelchair describes what anguish a polio victim causes among family members. The crippled boy cheers up his young friend and encourages him to receive the oral vaccine. The man lectures the two boys from his wheelchair on the seven steps to be taken to organize their neighborhood for the national polio vaccination campaign.

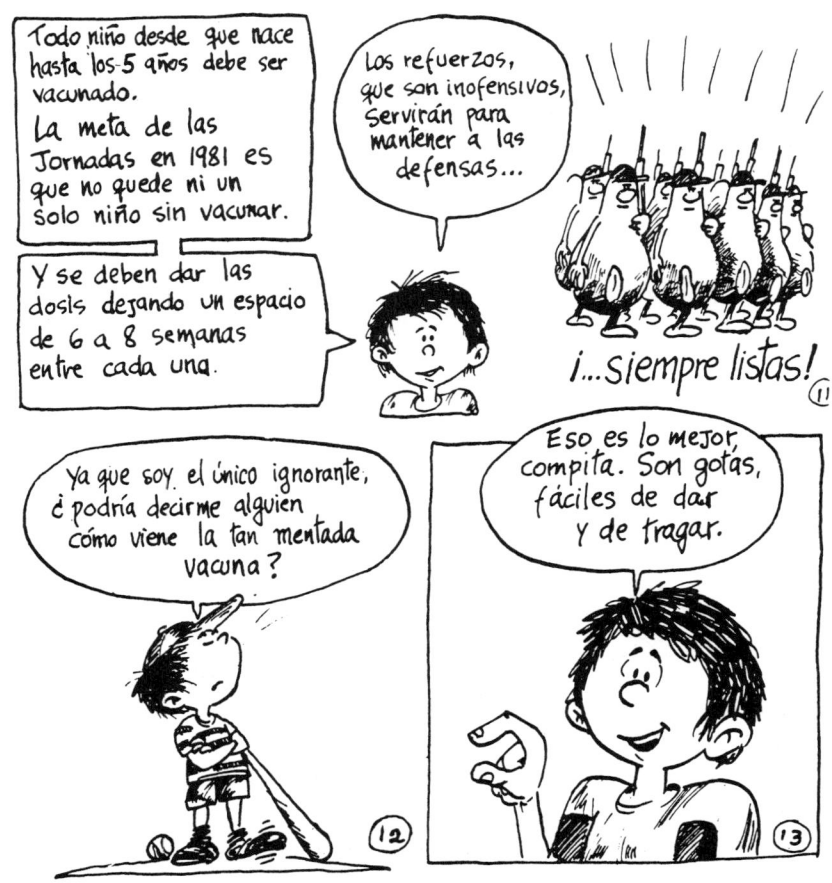

"Every child under 5 years of age should be vaccinated. The goal of the 1981 Popular Health Days is that no child will be left without the vaccine. And a space of six to eight weeks should be left between each dose." "The boosters, which really don't harm one, serve to maintain the defenses...ALWAYS READY."

"Since I am the only one who does not know, could someone tell me how this 'grand' vaccine is given?"

"That is the easy part, friend. They are drops which are easy to give and easy to take."

112 The Nicaraguan Revolution in Health

Pamphlet 5 El Sarampion (Measles). 4 pages.

   This booklet begins with a guide which directs the participants to read and answer two introductory questions, analyze the drawings and to discuss their answers after reading the pamphlet. The instruction discusses the prevalence of measles in Nicaragua, how the disease is transmitted and preventable through a vaccine. Prevention is compared to an invisible suit of armor. An analogy is drawn between the role of the Popular Militia and the vaccines in the defense of the body politic and of the human body.

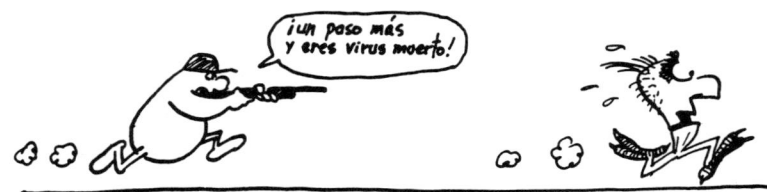

"One more step and you are a dead virus."

"Vaccination against measles will take place in the whole country during the Popular Health Campaigns."

"With the combined effort of the people now organized and the Ministry of Health, we will be able to quickly eliminate this disease from our country."

Pamphlet 6 <u>La</u> <u>Difteria</u>, <u>Tos</u> <u>Fernina</u>, <u>Tetano</u> (Diptheria, Whooping Cough, Tetanus). 12 pages.

The pamphlet discusses the etiology of the three diseases and the symptoms of each. Diptheria ("El Crup") is described as producing a poison which attacks the heart and the nervous system. The fish-like characterization of the crup germ illustrates how it flows through the bloodstream to the vital organs.

Whooping cough is represented by a snake-like virus which enters through the nasal passages and affects the throat, lungs and brain as the oxygen flow is impaired. Prevention is argued to be more desirable than a three to four month recuperation period.

The tetanus microbe is characterized as a centipede-like creature which attacks the nervous system. The symptoms of fever, muscular rigidity, and convulsions are depicted. Three folk beliefs ("creencias") as to the etiology of tetanus are debunked. Four measures are recommended to prevent tetanus infection in case of cuts and punctures and at the time of childbirth.

The final three pages are devoted to an explanation of the three vaccination series (DPT,DT,TT), care of the vaccine and how the temporary side effects of the vaccination are themselves indicative of the person's new immunity.

114   The Nicaraguan Revolution in Health

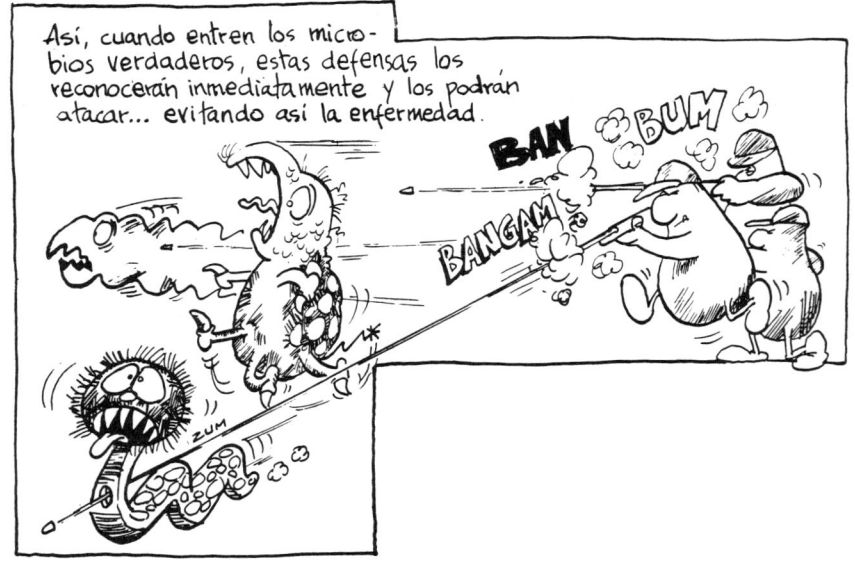

"So it is when the real microbes enter the body, these defenses will recognize them immediately and will be able to attack...and so avoid the disease."

Popular Health Pamphlets 115

Pamphlet 7 <u>El Agua</u> (Water). 8 pages.

The discussion guide poses several questions which address the importance of water, the general inaccessibility of potable water to the population and four ways in which water is contaminated. The final solution to water contamination is a safe water system in the cities and water wells in the rural countryside. The reality is other. Past monies for potable water systems were pocketed by the Somocistas.

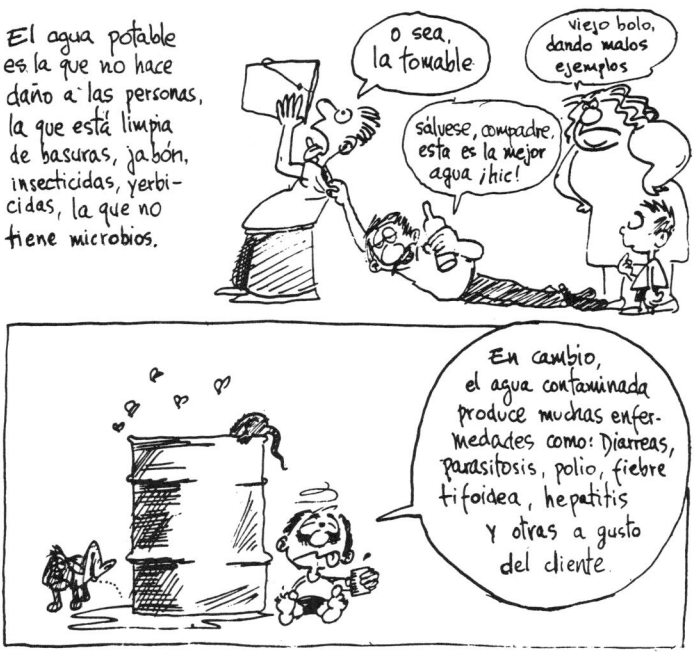

"Potable water is that which cannot harm people, that which is clean of garbage, soap, insecticides, pesticides and does not have microbes."

"Or in other words, that which is drinkable." "Save yourself, brother, this is the best water, hiccup!" "You old fool, you are setting a bad example."

"On the other hand, contaminated water produces many illnesses such as diarrhea, parasites, polio, fever, typhus, hepatitus and others made to order for the client."

Pamphlet 8 <u>La</u> <u>Higiene</u> <u>de</u> <u>Los</u> <u>Alimentos</u> (The Care of Food). 8 pages.

The theme of this discussion deals with "the enemies of food." The initial discussion focuses upon the enemies themselves. All foods have enemies. All foods are living things that die and begin to decompose. The "little animals" which feed upon decomposing food can make humans ill, if they are not killed before the food is eaten. The pig carries the most illnesses; fish decompose the fastest and chicken, the slowest. Fruits are exposed to other enemies such as the cockroach, flies and dust-borne germs.

These carriers of germs need to be eradicated. People who prepare food for others to eat need to be healthy themselves. Places of food preparation, such as slaughter houses, must be kept clean. The enemies of food can be defeated by personal and environmental cleanliness and by food preparation and storage.

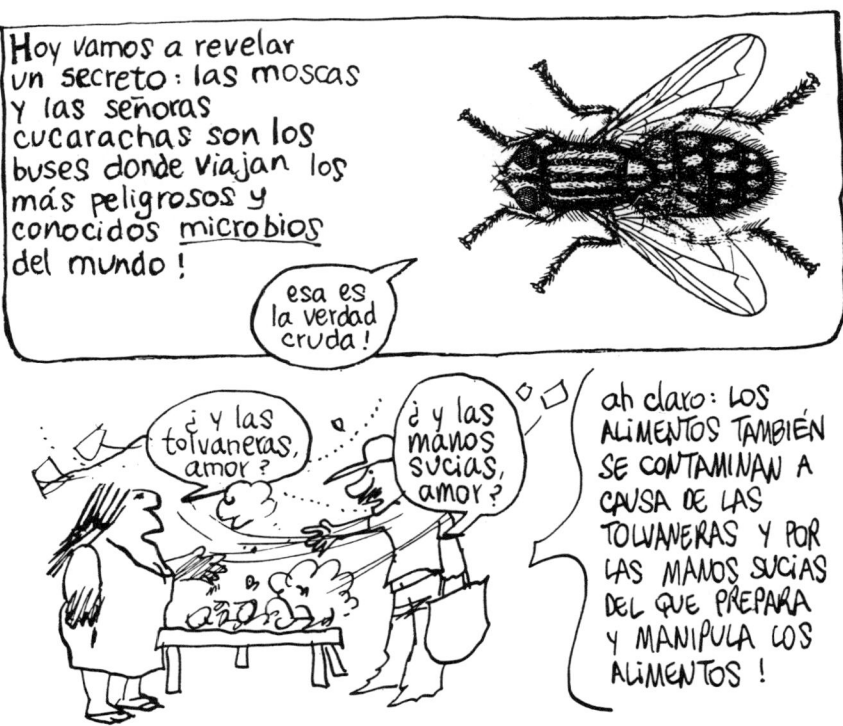

"Today we are going to reveal a secret: flies and the madame cockroach are the buses in which travel the most dangerous and well known microbes of the world."

"That is the gross truth."

"...and the dust, my love?"
"...and the dirty hands, love?"
"So. Foods also become contaminated by dust and the dirty hands of those who prepare and handle food."

Pamphlet 9 <u>Vida</u>, <u>Dolor</u>, y <u>Muerte</u> <u>de</u> <u>Los</u> <u>Dientes</u> (Life, Pain and Death of the Teeth). 12 pages.

After three introductory questions, there follows a discussion of why the teeth of Nicaraguans are on the average in such poor condition. The major cause is found in the characteristics of pre-revolutionary dentistry in Nicaragua: poor training of dentists, the maldistribution of dentists in the country and the fee-for-service and restorative focus of dentistry.

There follows an analysis of the new, low-cost, prevention program based upon (1) popular education as to the causes of dental disease, (2) prevention through brushing and (3) the application of a flouride mouthwash supervised by schoolteachers. Care of baby teeth is emphasized.

The pamphlet concludes with a discussion of a dental chart and a short explanation of gum disease and abscessed teeth. Two review questions are given.

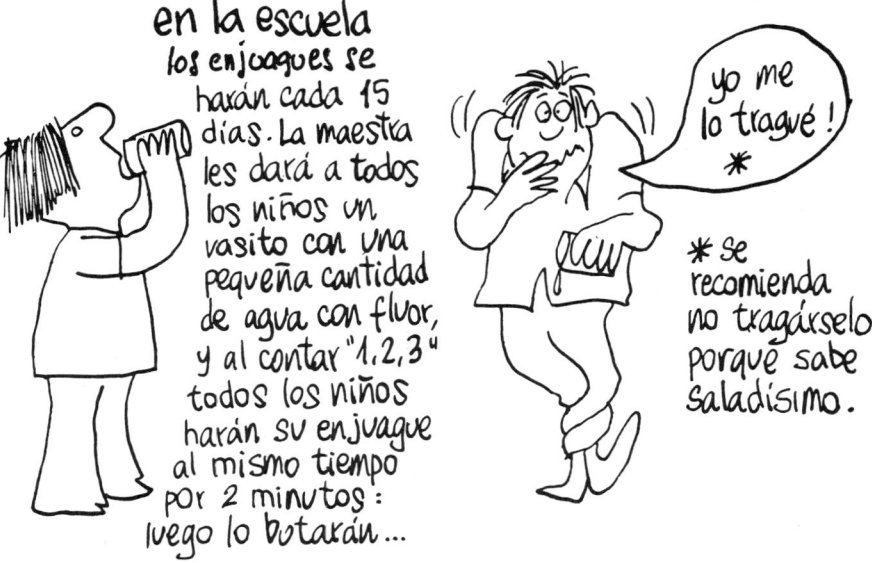

"The mouthwashes are given in school every 15 days. The teachers will give a little glass of water with a small amount of flouride to every student. After counting '1,2,3', all the children will gargle at the same time for two minutes and then spit out the mouthwash..." "I drank it! * Swallowing the solution is not recommended because it is very salty."

Pamphlet 10 <u>Basura</u> (Garbage). 8 pages.

Two questions, "What is garbage?" and "How do we become ill from garbage?" introduce the topic.

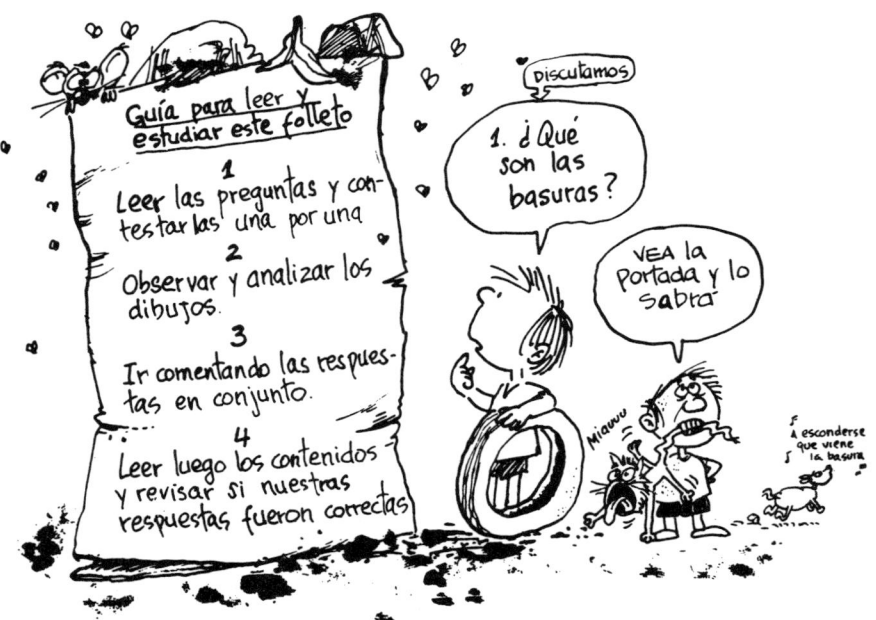

"Let's discuss. 1. What is garbage?"
"Look at the cover and and you will see."
"Let's hide. Here comes the garbage."

"Guide to read and study this pamphlet.
1. Read the questions and answer them one by one.
2. Look at and analyze the drawings.
3. Continue together commenting on your answers.
4. Then read the material and see if **your answers** were correct.

Popular Health Pamphlets   121

A discussion follows illustrating how garbage provides a home for disease-carrying animals such as flies, roaches and rats- -"the famous vectors." Garbage is shown to be the source of diseases such as diarrhea and parasitosis from which children have a right to be protected.

The discussion turns to four methods of garbage disposal. The practice of covering garbage is illustrated with an illusion to Somoza.

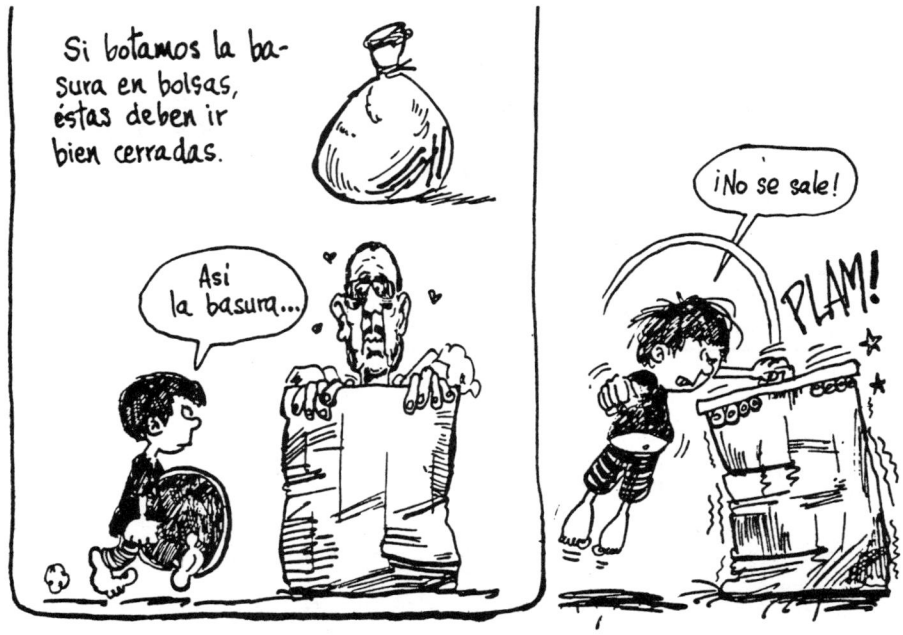

"If we throw out the garbage in bags, they should be well closed."

"In that way, the garbage does not get out."

[The discussion ends with a plan of action for the community.]

122   The Nicaraguan Revolution in Health

11. Los Vectores... Los Que? (The Vectors... The What?). 4 pages.

   Questions on vector identification and the illnesses transmitted begin the discussion. People are referred to the cover and asked to identify some twelve common vectors illustrated there. Two men discuss the major ways by which vectors transmit illnesses. Some carry the microbes on their bodies and others within their bodies, as in the case of the malaria mosquito.

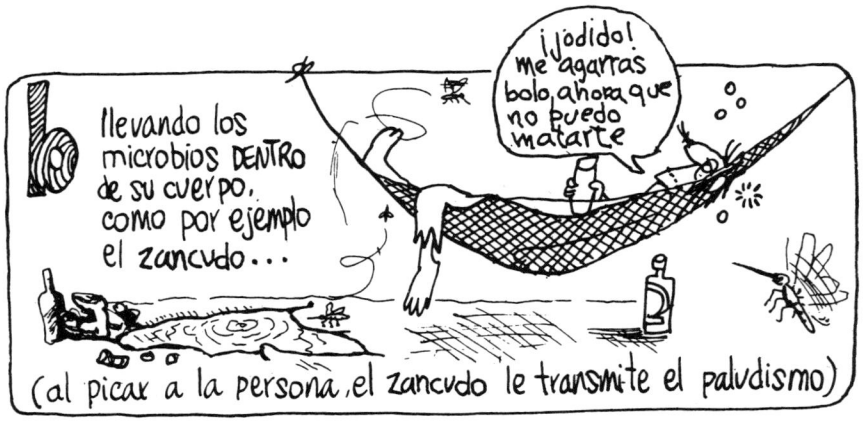

("The vectors can transmit diseases in two ways...) B. carrying the microbes within their body, as, for example, the mosquito..."

"Damm! You caught me drunk and I can't even kill you."

"The mosquito transmits malaria by biting the person."

   All disease vectors should be eliminated. Some diseases are not present in Nicaragua, but their vectors are and should be eliminated as well. Cleanliness is the weapon which humans can use to eliminate most vectors. If garbage and puddles are cleaned up, the area is then safe for children to play. They have a right to play and have fun in safe surroundings. The dialogue ends with a group discussion of what the community can do to eliminate vectors and prevent diseases.

Popular Health Pamphlets 123

Pamphlet 12 Que Hacer con las Excretas? (What to do with Excrements?). 8 pages.

Several questions and statistics begin the discussion of the enormity of the problem of human and animal waste disposal in Nicaragua after the Somoza dictatorship.

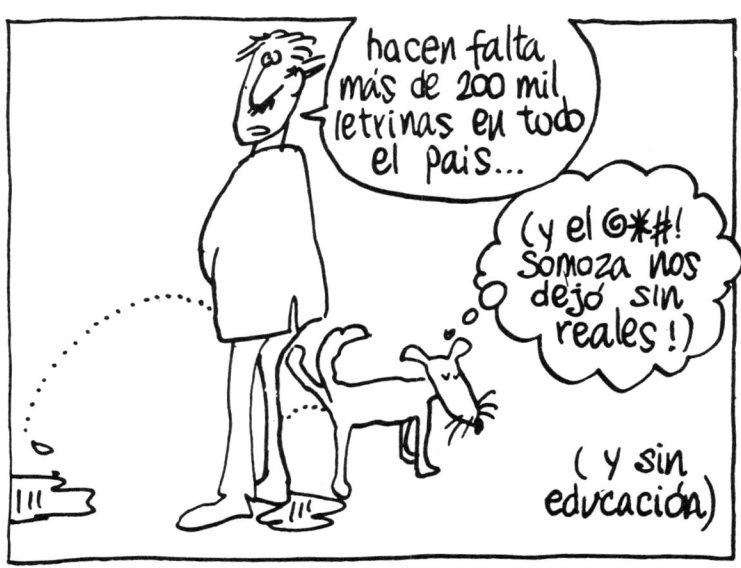

"More than 200,000 latrines are needed in the country...."
"(and that #*#* Somoza left us without money!)"
"(and without education)"

One section is devoted to explaining how and from what diseases humans become ill as a result of excrement. The discussion turns to how animal excrement can be controlled. The discussion of latrine building focuses upon the placement of the latrine relative to subterranean water supplies, the excavation and preparation of the pit, the construction of the platform, toilet seat and the building itself. The final section explains the use and care of latrines. Four summary questions initiate a discussion of the tasks that the members of the group need to address in order to control wastes in their community.

124 The Nicaraguan Revolution in Health

Pamphlet 13 <u>Ofensiva Contra La Malaria: Tratamiento Colectivo A Toda La Poblacion De Nicaragua - Octubre 1981</u> (The Final Offensive Against Malaria: Collective Treatment of the Entire Population of Nicaragua -- October 1981). 8 pages.

The pamphlet begins with an explanation that the first battle against malaria took place with the elimination of many of the breeding grounds of mosquitos. This final offensive involves a three day treatment of all Nicaraguans one year old and older with medicines which protect against infection. The medicines (colorquin and primaquin) are to be taken for three consecutive days. They protect the individual for twenty days. During that period of time the malaria carrying mosquito will die and the next generation will not have been infected. Since everyone will have taken the medicines, the new generation of mosquitos will have nowhere to infect themselves or others.

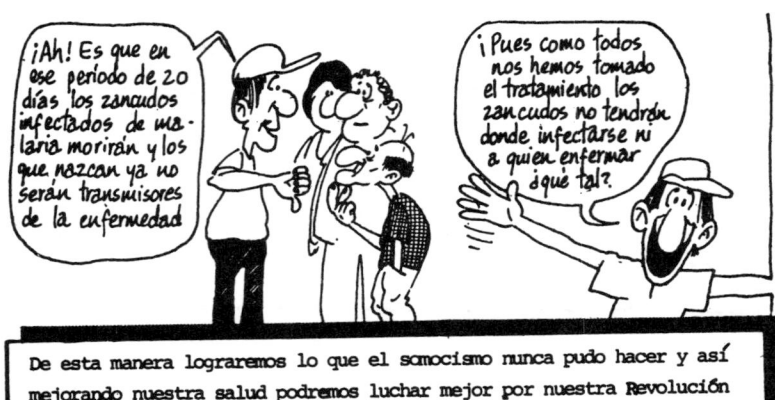

"Ah! The fact is that in a period of 20 days the mosquitos infected by malaria will die and those that are born will not be transmitters of the disease. Since all of us will have taken the medicines, the mosquitos will have nowhere to infect themselves nor make others ill. How about that?"

"In this way we accomplish what Somocismo was not able to do and improve our health so as to better struggle for the revolution. This accomplishment will bring prestige to our country inasmuch as no other nation in the world has ever done this."

Popular Health Pamphlets   125

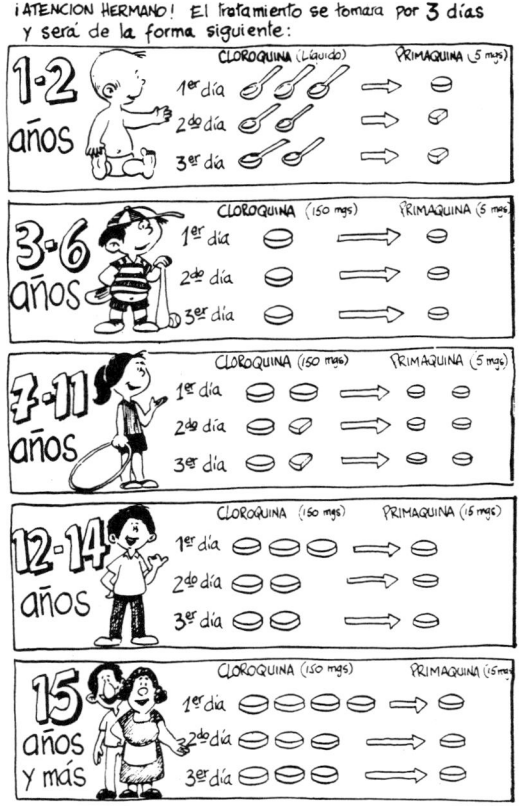

"Attention, Brother! The treatment will continue for three days and will be in the following manner:"

A short explanation of the possible side effects and recommended treatment follows. The pamphlet concludes with assurances that the medicines will not affect anyone be they healthy or ill or even pregnant. Children under one year of age are not treated unless they show signs and a blood test confirms that they have malaria. After the Campaign, anyone who shows signs of malaria should be taken to the malaria control office (ACEM).

Pamphlet 14 Las Causas de la Diarrea... Como Podemos Prevenirla ? (The Causes of Diarrea... How We Can Prevent It). 12 pages .

The study guide begins with an analysis of how and why class differences affect the incidence of diarrhea among children. Children whose parents enjoy good living conditions are less susceptible to diarrhea. Yet, diarrhea is the most common illness in Nicaragua and the one which causes most deaths to children under six years of age. The Revolution seeks to provide all Nicaraguans with access to the basic living conditions which encompass the work place, food, housing, a clean environment, education and health services.

The most common source of diarrhea is contact with the microbes and parasites which live in human and animal excrement. These disease carriers find their way into streams after rains and into the air during the windy, dry season. Dirty hands and unwashed fruit can also carry the germs.

The principle complication of diarrhea is dehydration which can kill a child in a few hours due to loss of fluids. The symptoms of the dehydrated child are described. There follow the "12 Commandments" which, if followed, can prevent diarrhea. They include (1) breastfeeding during the child's first year, (2) daily garbage disposal in the home, (3) use and care of the latrine, (4) hand washing before meal preparation, (5) boiling water, (6) washing of fruits and vegetables, (7) boiling baby bottles, (8) care of children's toys, (9) proper food storage, (10) coralling of animals, (11) cutting fingernails short and washing of hands before eating and (12) keeping healthy children away from children with diarrhea.

Prevention plus efforts to reduce economic inequalities will decrease illness and death due to diarrhea.

Popular Health Pamphlets 127

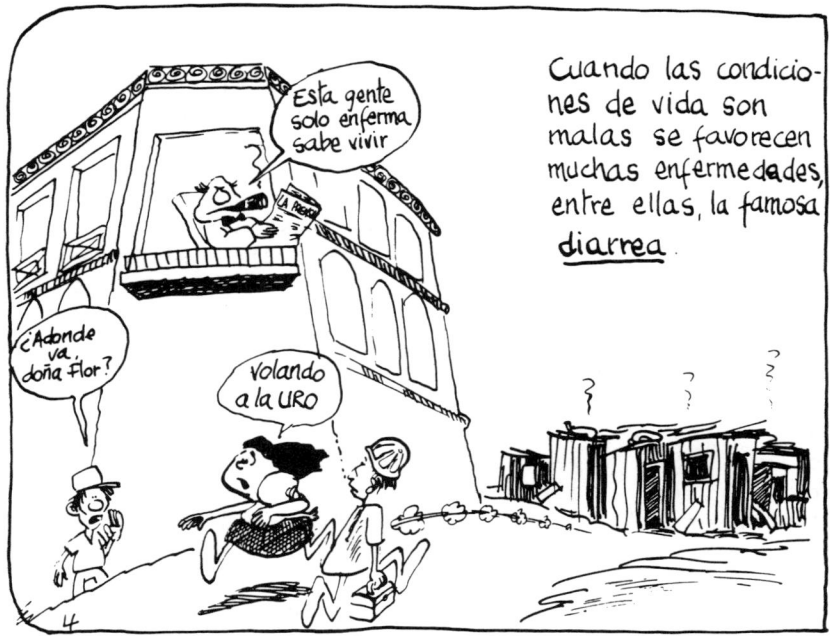

"When the conditions of life are poor, any number of illnesses flourish, among them the famous diarrhea."

"Where are you going, Miss Flor?" "I'm running to the URO (oral rehydration post)."

"These people only know how to get sick."

Pamphlet 15 <u>Como</u> <u>Tratar</u> <u>la</u> <u>Diarrea</u> (How to Treat Diarrhea). 8 pages.

A nurse introduces the discussion pamphlet with the question, "What are the oral rehydration units (URO)"? A mother explains that these are the means that the Ministry of Health provide so that children do not die from dehydration. For the URO to be effective three steps must be followed. Diarrhetic children must be taken immediately to the neighborhood Oral Rehydration Unit Post. There must be a follow-up at home and finally, the community must constantly educate itself to the problem.

Mothers are advised to expect that children will pass much of the URO that they receive. More liquid will stay in the body than will be lost. Like a jar with a hole in it, the water level will be maintained as long as more water is added than is lost. If the child vomits, one should wait twenty minutes, give him air and repeat the URO in small doses. After three to six hours the child should be rehydrated.

The discussion next turns to the preparation of the URO through seven steps. Mothers are instructed to boil the water before adding the URO salts. The child should be given the mixture only when it is cooled and so avoid vomiting. No sugar should be added to the URO salts.

Five suggestions are made as to feeding a child with diarrhea. "To leave the intestine rest" is a popular custom, but it is not correct. If the child is breastfeeding, it should continue to take the mother's milk, but no other. Certain local vegetables, rice, toasted crackers, and tortillas can be given to avoid weight loss and malnutrition. After a time, children can be returned to cow's milk and to other foods. The booklet concludes with three points. Children with diarrhea usually only need the URO. They should continue eating and above all, parents should work to prevent future incidents of the illness.

Popular Health Pamphlets 129

Pamphlet 16   El Mejor Alimento   (The Best Food).   16 pages.

   Three general questions introduce the topic.
"Why do some women breastfeed and others not?"
"Why is breastmilk superior to other kinds of milk?"
"What precautions should be taken before giving the breast?"
   Nine advantages of breastfeeding are discussed. They include the prevention of malnutrition; protection against diarrhea and respiratory illness; reduction of colic; practicality over baby bottles and formula; emotional bonding between mother and child; ability of breastmilk to be kept in a bottle without refrigeration so that the child can feed while the mother is at work; reduction of risk of breast cancer; normalization of the womb after birth; the economic savings of breastmilk for the family and for the country.
   The fact is that the custom of breastfeeding is on the wane in Nicaragua as in other countries of the world.

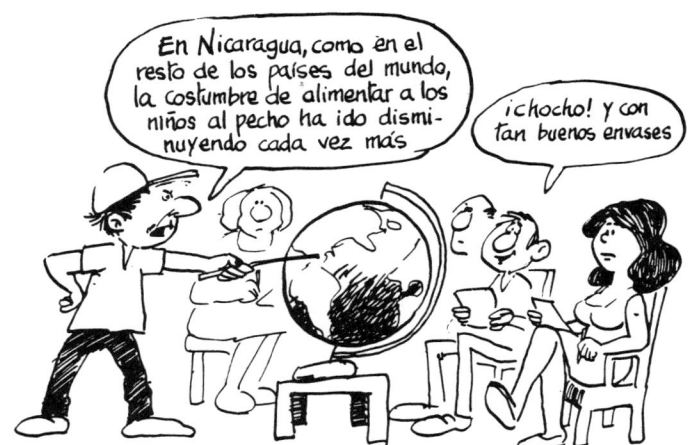

"In Nicaragua, as in the rest of the world, the custom of breastfeeding has been steadily on the decline."
"Wow! And with such fine containers."

Four reasons are given for the decline. They include the influence in the marketplace of the corporate producers of infant formula, the susceptibility of physicians and nurses to their influence and those of some parents, social pressure and several incorrect beliefs pertaining to breastfeeding.

Seven common misconceptions or beliefs ("creencias") are critiqued. They include the belief that the first days' breastmilk is of insufficient quantity and quality; that mothers who are malnourished produce poor milk; that some breasts produce little milk and quickly dry up; that when children cry, it is because they have not received enough milk; that if breasts are small, they cannot produce enough milk; that when mothers become angry, their milk becomes bad; that when a mother is ill, she should not breastfeed. The discussion shows why the reverse of each of these beliefs is true. The conclusion is that more mothers should give the breast so that when their children grow up, they will do the same with their children.

Seven steps are given to enhance the act of breastfeeding. The discussion is concluded with the statement that breastfeeding is a revolutionary obligation which the community should support. In this way children will enjoy their right to good food and avoid malnutrition. The fact that mothers are part of the revolutionary process does not have to detract from breastfeeding.

Pamphlet 17 <u>La</u> <u>Alimentacion</u> <u>del</u> <u>Nino</u> en <u>el</u> <u>Primer</u> <u>Ano</u> <u>de</u> <u>Vida</u> (The Feeding of Children in Their First Year).
12 pages.

    The group is asked to reflect on the consequences of the fact that 67 out of every 100 children in Nicaragua are malnourished. Malnutrition dates from the time of Somoza and the unjust distribution of wealth which characterized that period. In conjunction with the efforts of the Revolution to rectify that legacy, mothers can take concrete steps to improve the diet of their children. Breastmilk is itself the best food for a child in its first year. In the first two months breastmilk can be supplemented with boiled water. In the third month the child can be given juices mixed with water. In the fourth month pureed chicken, liver and vegetables can be added to the diet. In the fifth month pureed egg yolk, rice, beans, corn derivatives, cooked yucca, bread and crackers can supplement breastmilk. In the sixth through ninth month noodles, cheese, fish and ground meats are appropriate. In the ninth month the child should sit at the family table and gradually be weaned.
    The discussion next turns to eight preventive measures which one should take to insure that when the child feeds, he does not become ill. The discussion ends with a question, "What will we do to multiply this knowledge?"

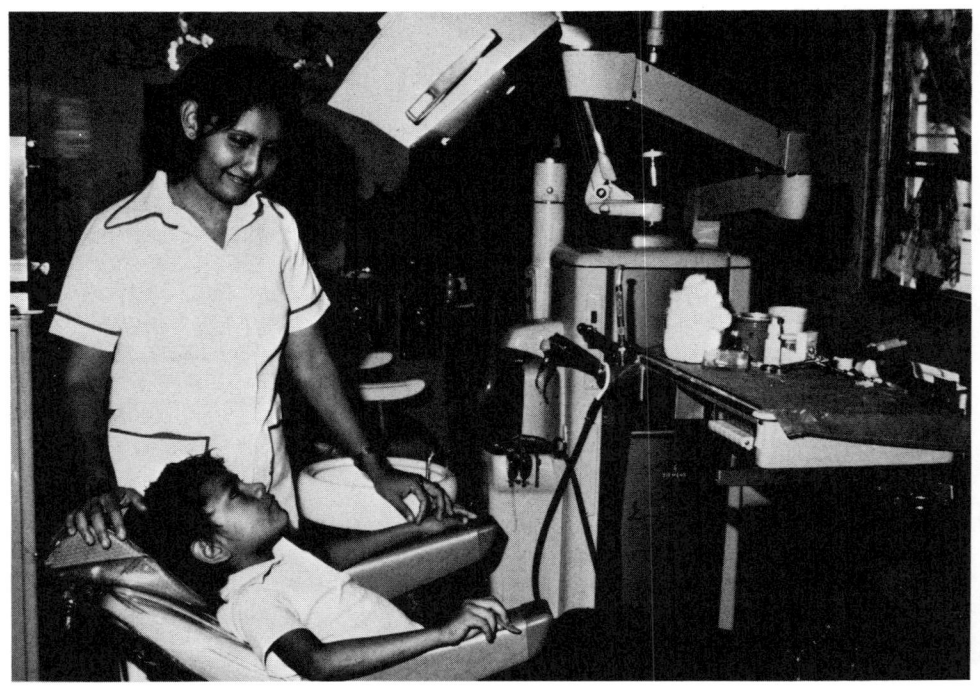

This dental hygienist (with her son) is part of the national effort to improve dental care.

Appendix B
POPULAR HEALTH DOCUMENTS

A series of documents on various health themes, published in 1981, were intended to form part of a training manual for the Health Multipliers and Brigadistas.

Manual del Brigadista Popular de Salud: Jornadas Populares de Salud (Manual of the Popular Health Brigadista). 32 pages, 1981.

This is a training manual for both Multipliers and Brigadistas. It begins with an overview of the health problems inherited from the Somoza era. The five Popular Health Days planned for 1981 are then described. The coordinating bodies at each level have a corresponding organizational component. Volunteers at the Departmental level are organized into "Health Brigades", into "columns" at the Municipal (county) level, into "columns" at the Zonal level, and into "squadrons" at the neighborhood or rural village level. The coordinating bodies are made up of the National Popular Health Commission and the Ministry of Health at the National level and the Popular Health Councils and Ministry officials at each of the other levels. The Manual turns to a description of the duties of the Popular Trainer ("El Capacitador Popular"). This person is the Health Educator for the Ministry of Health at the Municipal level. He/she is responsible for the training of the Health Multipliers who in turn will train 20 Health Brigadistas each. The Manual lists six organizational and educational functions for the Multipliers and 18 specific tasks related to those functions. The Manual lists 12 functions for the Popular Health Brigadista and 16 tasks related to those functions. The next topic deals with the dynamics of the educational process which the Brigadista will employ in training people in the neighborhood for the Popular Health Campaigns. The discussion revolves around the objectives of the group discussions and how to coordinate a group discussion using the popular health pamphlets. Further guidance is provided in the use of teaching techniques other than the pamphlets. These include the "newspaper billboard," charts and the sociodrama. Several group dynamics techniques are offered. These include "personal introduction games," "recreational games," and "concentration games." The Manual concludes with a discussion of the technical aspects of each of the five planned Popular Health Days. Each Campaign is discussed in terms of the objectives, preparation and execution.

Documento No.1: Primera Movilizacion Vacunacion Antipolio (Document No 1.: The First Antipolio Vaccination Mobilization). 24 pages, March 1981.

This document is a discussion leader's manual. The first theme deals with two content areas. The first is that of vaccinations: the need, the types of vaccines and the illnesses that they prevent. The discussion of each item is referenced to the appropriate Popular Health Pamphlet. An analogy is drawn between the role of the Popular Militia and the vaccines in the defense of the body politic and the human body. The second theme deals with the polio vaccination and provides the Health Brigadista with questions and examples to facilitate discussion of that Popular Health Pamphlet.

The Manual turns to a discussion of the group dynamics which facilitate the discussion of the above content areas, the location and organization of the vaccination posts, care of the vaccine, record keeping and evaluation procedures. The Health Information and Evaluation System is explained at length.

Documento No.2: Segunda Movilizacion Limpieza Ambiental (Document No 2.: Second Environmental Cleanup Mobilization). 14 pages, May 1981.

This document was issued to assist in the organization at the local level of the 2nd Environmental Cleanup of 1981. Thirteen tasks are outlined for the neighborhood communities and the Health Brigadistas. The narrative details each task which is accompanied by an illustrative drawing. The captions are reproduced below to provide an organizational flow chart of the mobilization.

1. Program Activities
2. Workshops
3. Community Education
4. Organization of Neighborhood "Squadrons"
5. The Environmental Survey
6. Preparation of Work Assignments
7. County-level Coordination Meetings
8. Community Motivation
9. Execution of Cleanup Tasks
10. Execution of Beautification Tasks
11. Evaluation and Information Tasks
12. Community Recognition Meetings
13. Follow-up Strategy Meetings

The appendix contains an organizational chart, a calendar of events including workshops, dates of vaccinations, home visits of children not vaccinated and evaluations, a series of sample forms and instructions, the format for the workshops, recommendations for the preservation of the vaccine and evaluation procedures.

Documento No.3: Movilizacion Nacional Antimalarica (Document No. 3.: National Antimalaria Campaign). 16 pages, June 1981.

The Document begins with a cost/benefit analysis of the National Malaria Control Program (SNEM) during the period 1958-1980. During that 22-year period more than one billion cordovas were expended in the control and eradication of malaria. Yet, the program failed to have a major impact on the prevalence of the disease in Nicaragua. In 1980 the value of production lost due to malaria illness was about $51 million cordovas. Salary loss due to sick days was about $22,600,000 cordovas. Hospitalization costs were $16,300,000 cordovas. Over five years this would represent a projected loss of $ 90,201,000 cordovas. Malaria Program costs for the period 1980-1985 are pegged at $250,000,000 cordovas. The traditional Malaria Control Program is not cost effective nor has it been effective in preventing the human suffering occasioned by the disease.

Initial efforts during the Literacy Campaign of 1981 to control breeding grounds of mosquitos resulted in a lessening of the reported cases from 35,000 expected that year to 25,465 cases. The stage is now set for the first National Popular Campaign to control malaria. There follows a detailed description of fourteen tasks necessary to carry out the Anti-malaria mobilization.

Vacunacion Anti-polio 1982 (Anti-polio Vaccination 1982). 31 pages.

Movilizacion : Antipolio (2nd Dosis) DPT y Antisarampionosa
(Mobilization: Antipolio [2nd dosis] DPT y Antimeasles). 14 pages.

In 1982 a second series of health documents was published. The first was a popular training manual for the Second Antipolio Vaccination programed for February 7 (1st dosis), March 21 (2nd dosis) and May 9 (3rd dosis). In conjunction with the training manual for Health Educators and Multipliers, a second pamphlet was prepared for the Health Brigadistas in charge of the vaccination posts. In both cases the primary emphasis is less on the epidemiology of the disease and more on the organizational demands of the mobilization. Included are such items as the preparation of the vaccination posts, ways to motivate the community, the census of children at risk, the care of the medicines, record keeping, evaluation and follow-up. The coordinating unit is the Local Antipolio Committee made up of the Barrio Committees (Comite de Direccion Zonal), Ministry of Health personnel, representatives of AMNLAE and the CDS. The members divide up the various tasks among them. These include the designation of one post for every 250 children. The second task is to organize the workshops so that Multipliers, Brigadistas and Health personnel each understand their task. After the workshops, the barrio is divided up into neighborhood "squadrons" ("escuadras") for the purpose of census and promotional activities. Procedures are given for the day of the vaccination. The number of children vaccinated are reported to the Local Committee, but the Brigadista keeps the forms for the second and third vaccinations. Evaluations are carried out at the local, county, departmental and national levels.

There follows a discussion of the second and third phases based upon the experience of the first phase. Newborns and children not vaccinated in the first phase are to be noted. After the third phase, a final report is sent to the County-level Coordinating Commission. Evaluation and follow-up procedures are discussed.

Saneamiento Ambiental: Agua, Excretas, Vectores y Basuras (Environmental Health: Water, Wastes, Vectors and Garbage). 32 pages.

This manual begins with a discussion of water contamination. Diarrhetic diseases are seen as typical of underdeveloped countries, especially those which have dictatorial governments. The World Health Organization estimates that three out of four hospital beds around the world are taken by people suffering from water-borne diseases. Nine ways that well water may become contaminated are illustrated. Contamination of other water sources is discussed: pools, piped water, surface water and rain water. Definitions and illustrations are given of potable water, purification, boiling and filtration. Instructions are provided as how to protect wells, pools, piped water and surface water from contamination. Five methods of storing water are discussed. The problem of waste water and mosquito breeding is analyzed.

The next part deals with the problem of human and animal waste disposal. Contamination, control and prevention are discussed. Extended instructions are given for the construction and care of the latrine.

The final part deals with vectors and garbage disposal. Special care is taken to analyze how mosquito breeding can be controlled. The discussion evolves around the proper disposal of waste water, elimination of standing water, spraying and chemical control of standing water with the use of a porous container of insecticide ("abate").

Manual de Primeros Auxilios (First Aid Manual).
44 pages.

This manual was developed to be used in the training of Health Multipliers and Brigadistas during the latter part of 1982. The contents address (1) a definition of First Aid, (2) signs of life, (3) wounds, (4) classification and treatment of wounds, (5) shock, (6) trauma, (7) fractures, (8) treatment of fractures, (9) dislocations and strains, (10) suffocation, (11) resuscitation, (12) burns, (13) rescue and transportation, (14) bandages.

REFERENCES

REFERENCES

Adams, R.
1970 Brokers and Career Mobility Systems in the Structure of Complex Societies. <u>Southwestern Journal of Anthropology</u> 24:315-327.

Anderson, R, B. Smedly and O.W. Anderson.
1970 Medical Care Use in Sweden and the United States: A Comparative Analysis of Systems and Behavior. Chicago: Center for Health Administration. Research Series No. 27.

Assmann, H.
1981 Nicaragua: Triunfo de la Alfabetizacion. San Jose, Costa Rica: Ministerio de Educacion (Nicaragua) y Departamento Ecumenico de Investigaciones.

Baer, H. A.
1982 On the Political Economy of Health. <u>Medical Anthropology Newsletter</u> 14:1.

<u>Barricada</u>
1983 Nicaragua es Modelo de Salud para America Latina. Wednesday, July 13, p.14.

Booth, J. A.
1985 The End and the Beginning: The Nicaraguan Revolution. Second Edition. Boulder, Colo.: Westview Press.

Bossert, T.
1982 Health Care in Revolutionary Nicaragua. In Nicaragua in Revolution, T. Walker, editor. New York: Praeger, pp.259-272.

1984 Nicaraguan Health Policy: The Dilemma of Success. Medical Anthropology Quarterly 15(3):73-74.

1985 Health Policy. Nicaragua: The First Five Years. T.W. Walker, ed. New York: Praeger, pp. 347-365.

CIERA (Centro de Investigaciones y Estudios de la Reforma Agraria)
1982 3 Anos de Reforma Agraria. Managua:CIERA.

Collins, J.
1982 What Difference Could a Revolution Make? Food and Farming in the New Nicaragua. San Francisco: Food First.

Confederacion Universitaria Centroamericana
1981 Preproyecto de Evaluacion del Sector Salud en Nicaragua con Enfasis en el Desarrollo de las Formas Participativas que se Dan a Nivel de las Organizaciones Populares. San Jose: Programa Centroamericano de Ciencias de la Salud.

Danielson, R.
1975 The Cuban Health Area and Polyclinic: Organizational Focus in an Emerging System. Inquiry. Supplement to Volume XII, June 1975, pp. 86-102.

1979 Cuban Medicine, New Brunswick: Transaction Books.

DeMiguel, J. M.
1975 A Framework for the Study of National Health Systems. Inquiry. Supplement to Volume XII, June 1975, pp.10-24.

DECOPS/MINSA
1982 Las Jornadas Populares de Salud. Unpublished report. Ministerio de Sauld. p.1.

DECOPS/MINSA
1983 Estrategia de Capacitacion Popular en la Atencion Primaria de Salud en Nicaragua. Managua: Ministerio de Salud, Republica de Nicaragua.

Donahue, J. M.
1981 Health Delivery in Rural Bolivia. Health in the Andes. J. Bastien and J. M. Donahue, eds. Washington, D.C.: The American Anthropological Association.

1983 The Politics of Health Care in Nicaragua Before and After the Revolution of 1979. Human Organization 42(3):264-272.

1984 Studying the Transition to Socialism in the Nicaraguan Health System. Medical Anthropology Quarterly 15(3):70-71.

ECLA (U.N. Economic Commission for Latin America)
1979 Nicaragua: Repercusiones Economicas de los Acontecimientos Politicos Recientes. E/CEPAL/G.1279 (December 29).

Elling, R.
1980 Cross-National Study of Health Systems: Political Economies and Health Care. New Brunswick: Transaction Books.

Elling, R. H. and H. Kerr
1975 Selection of Contrasting National Health Systems for In-Depth Study. Inquiry. Supplement to Volume XII, June, 1975, pp. 25-40.

Ellsberg, M. C.
1982 Educacion y Participacion Popular en Salud. Revista Centroamericana de Ciencias de la Salud 23:145-161.

1983 Trail Blazing on the Atlantic Coast. Science For the People 15(6):14-19.

England, R.
1978 More Myths in International Health Planning. American Journal of Public Health 68(2):153-159.

Escalona, M.
n.d. "Participacion Popular en Cuba." Mimeo.

Escudero, Jose Carlos
1980 Starting from Year One: The Politics of Health in Nicaragua. International Journal of Health Services 10(4):647-656.

Fanon, F.
1963 The Wretched of the Earth. New York: Grove Press.

Firth, R.
1963 Elements of Social Organization. Boston: Beacon Press.

Freidson, E.
1970 Professional Dominance. New York: Atherton Press.

1984 The Changing Nature of Professional Control. The Annual Review of Sociology 10:1-20.

Freire, P.
1970 Pedagogy of the Oppressed. New York: Herder and Herder.

1974 Educacion Popular: Su Dimension Politicia. Lima: Editorial Tarea.

1978 Pedagogy in Progress: The Letters to Guinea-Bissau. New York:Seabury.

Gamer, R. E.
1982 The Developing Nations: A Comparative Perspective. Boston: Allyn and Bacon.

Garfield, R. M.
1985 Health and the War Against Nicaragua, 1981-84. Journal of Public Health Policy 6(1):116-131.

Garfield, R.M. and D.C. Halperin
1983 Health Care in Nicaragua. New England Journal of Medicine 309:193.

Garfield, R. and E. Taboada
1984 Health Service Reforms in Revolutionary Nicaragua. American Journal of Public Health 74(10):1133-1144.

Garfield R. and S. Vermund
1983a Malaria Control in Nicaragua: Health Promotion Through a Mass Drug Administration Campaign. Columbia University, Department of Epidemiology. Mimeo.

1983b Changes in Malaria Incidence After Mass Drug Administration in Nicaragua. Lancet August 27, pp.500-503.

Greaves, T. C.
1982 The "dependencias" of Health, Illness and Death in Two Andean Labor Contexts. Paper presented at the 81st Annual Meeting of the American Anthopological Association. Washington, DC.

Halperin, D. C. and R. Garfield
1982 Developments in Health Care in Nicaragua: Special Report. New England Journal of Medicine 307:388-392.

Haug, M.
1973 Deprofessionalization: An Alternative Hypothesis for the Future. Sociological Review Monographs 20:195-211.

1975 The Deprofessionalization of Everyone? Sociological Focus 3:197-213.

1977 Computer Technology and the Obsolescence of the Concept of Profession. In Work and Technology, M.R. Haug and J. Dofny, editors. Beverly Hills:Sage, pp. 215-228.

Heath, D. B. and R. Adams (eds.)
1974 Contemporary Cultures and Societies of Latin America. New York:Random House.

Heiby, J. R.
1981 Low Cost Health Delivery Systems: Lessons from Nicaragua. American Journal of Public Health 71(5):514-519, also published in World Health Forum 3(1):27-29 (1982).

Helms, M.
1982 Nicaragua: the Society and Its Environment. In Nicaragua: A Country Profile. James D. Rudolph, ed. Department of the Army. Washington, D.C.: Government Printing Office.

Holland B., J.Davis and L. Gangloff
1973 Syncrisis: The Dynamics of Health XI: Nicaragua. Washington, DC: U.S. Government Printing Office.

INCAP (Instituto de Nutricion para Centroamerica y Panama)
1966 Evaluacion Nutricional de la Poblacion de Centro America y Panama. Nicaragua.

INCAP/CDC (Institute of Nutrition for Central America and Panama and Center for Disease Control)
1971 Nutritional Evaluation of the Population of Central America and Panama: Regional Summary. Washington: DHEW Publication No. (HSM) 72-8120 p. 45.

INSSBI (Instituto Nicaraguense de Seguridad Social y Bienestar)
1984 Repercusion del Terrorismo de Estado de la Administracion Reagan en la Vida del Pueblo Nicaraguense. Managua: Comite Nacional de Emergencia.

Jara, O.
1981 Educacion Popular: La Dimension Educativa de la Accion Politica: Reflexiones Sobre la Educacion Popular Desde el Contexto de la Revolucion Sandinista. Panama: CEASPA.

Junta de Gobierno de Reconstruccion Nacional, Republica de Nicaragua
n.d. La Salud en Nicaragua Antes y Despues del Triunfo de la Revolucion. Managua: Ministerio de Salud.

Keyzer, B. de and J. Ulate
1980 Educacion, Participacion en Salud e Ideologia: Nicaragua Pasado y Presente. Revista Centroamericana de Ciencias de las Salud Numero 17.

Korten, D. C.
1982 Organizing for Rural Development: A Learning Process. Development Digest 20(2):3-30.

Lampton, D. M.
1974 Health, Conflict and the Chinese Political System. Michigan Papers in Chinese Studies, No. 18. Ann Arbor: The University of Michigan.

Miller, V.
1985 Between Struggle and Hope: The Nicaraguan Literacy Crusade. Boulder, Colo.: Westview.

Millett, R.
1977 The Guardians of the Dynasty: A History of the U.S. Created Guardia Nacional de Nicaragua and the Somoza Family. Maryknoll, New York: Orbis Books.

MSP (Ministry of Public Health, Republic of Nicaragua)
 1975 Politicas, Estrategias y Organizacion de la Division de Educacion para la Salud. Managua: Ministerio de Salud Publica. Abril de 1975. Mimeo.

MSP-PLANSAR (Ministry of Public Health/ Plan for Rural Sanitation)
 1977 Informe Sobre la Situacion Actual de la Entidad Ejecutora de PLANSAR y Propuesta para el Desarrollo de su Capacidad Operativa. Nicaragua, Agosto de 1977. Mimeo.

MINSA (Ministry of Health, Republic of Nicaragua)
 1980a Aportes para el Analysis Historico de la Educacion y La Participacion Popular en Salud. Managua: Direccion de Educacion y Communicacion Popular en Salud.

 1980b Primer Aniversario del Sistema Nacional Unico de Salud. Boletin No. 15. 14 de Agosto. Managua.

 1980c Educacion Popular en Salud: Lineamientos Generales. Managua: Division de Comunicacion y Educacion Popular en Salud (DECOPS).

 1981a Educacion y Participacion en Salud. Managua.

 1981b Informe 1980. Managua: Ministerio de Salud, Republica de Nicaragua.

 1982a Principios y Politicas del Gobierno de Nicaragua. El Sistema Nacional Unico de Salud: Tres Anos de Revolucion 1979-1982. Managua: Ministerio de Salud, Republica de Nicaragua. pp. 1-12, 53-57.

 1982b Plan Integral de Actividades del Area de Salud-- Libro Rojo y Negro. Managua: Ministerio de Salud, Republica de Nicaragua.

 1982c Las Jornadas Populares de Salud. Unpublished report. Managua: Division de Comunicacion y Educacion Popular en Salud (DECOPS). Managua: Ministerio de Salud, Republica de Nicaragua.

146 The Nicaraguan Revolution in Health

MINSA (Ministry of Health, Republic of Nicaragua)
  1982d El Sistema Nacional Unico de Salud: Tres Anos de Revolucion 1979-1982. Managua: Ministerio de Salud, Republica de Nicaragua.

  1983 Plan de Salud 1983. Managua: Ministerio de Salud, Republica de Nicaragua.

  1984 Plan de Salud 1984. Managua: Ministerio de Salud, Republica de Nicaragua.

  1985 Lineamientos de Politicas de Salud: Plan de Actividades 1985. Managua: Ministerio de Salud, Republica de Nicaragua

  n.d. Guia de Programacion de Actividades para el Desarrollo de la Estrategia de Atencion Primaria a Nivel de Region y Area de Salud. Managua: Ministerio de Salud, Republica de Nicaragua.

MINSA/DECOPS (Ministry of Health/Division of Education and Popular Communication in Health)
  1982 Las Jornadas Populares de Salud. Managua. Mimeo.

MINSA/CONSEJO POPULAR DE SALUD - REGION IV (Ministry of Health, Popular Health Council-Region IV)
  1984 El Papel de los Consejos Populares de Salud en las Jornadas Populares de Salud. 1er Congreso Nacional JPS "Julio Cesar Martinez Obando." Managua: Ministerio de Salud.

MINSA/REGION II (Ministry of Health/Region II)
  1984 Evaluacion de la Region de Salud. Leon: Ministerio de Salud, Republica de Nicaragua.

MIPLAN/MINSA (Ministry of Planning/Ministry of Health)
  1981 Estrategias de Atencion Primaria de la Sauld en la Republica de Nicaragua. Managua: Ministerio de Planificacion y Ministerio de Salud, Republica de Nicaragua.

Montis, M. de, H. Molina, I. Tercero T., C. Jarquin G., H. Jaramillo H., J. M. Bisso, N. Garcia M., R. Capote M.
  1981 Estrategias de Atencion Primaria de la Salud en la Republica de Nicaragua. Managua: Ministerio de Planificacion (MIPLAN) y Ministerio de Salud (MINSA). Mimeo.

Mott, B.J.
1974 Politics and International Planning. Social Science and Medicine 8:271-274.

Navarro, V.
1976 Medicine Under Capitalism. New York: Prodist.

1977 Social Security and Medicine in the USSR: a Marxist Critique. Lexington, MA: Lexington Books.

1980 Workers and Community Participation and Democratic Control in Cuba. International Journal of Health Services 10(2):197-216.

n.d. "El subdesarrollo de la salud o la salud del subdesarrollo." Cuadernos de la Salud, CSUCA. San Jose, Costa Rica.

New, P. K.
1984 Primary Health Care in the People's Republic of China: A March Backward? Paper presented at the annual meetings of the American Anthropological Association. Denver, CO, November 15.

New, P.K., R.M. Hessler and P.B. Cater
1973 Consumer Participation and Public Accountability Anthropological Quarterly 46:196-213.

New, P. K and M. L New
1975 The Links Between Health and the Political Structure in New China. Human Organization 34(3):237-251.

Ortega, Daniel
1985 Daniel y los Medicos de Nicaragua: Problemas, Medidas y Compromiso. Managua: Direccion de Informacion y Prensa de la Presidencia de la Republica.

PAHO (Pan American Health Organization)
1979 Condiciones de Salud del Nino en las Americas. Publicacion No. 381. Washington: Organizacion Panamericana de Salud.

Pechersky, G.
1981 La Participacion de los Organismos de Masas en las Acciones del Sector Salud en El Departamento de Leon, Nicaragua. Leon: Ministero de Salud. Mimeo.

PRACS (Programa Rural de Accion Comunitaria)
1977 Definicion del Colaborador Rural de Salud (C.R.S.) Nicaragua. Mimeo.

Rifkin, S.B.
1973 Public Health in China -- Is the Experience Relevant to Other Less Developed Nations? Social Science and Medicine 7:249-257.

Rius (Eduardo del Rio)
1976 Marx for Beginners. New York: Pantheon.

1976 Lenin for Beginners. New York: Pantheon.

1982 Nicaragua for Beginners. New York: Writers and Readers Publishing, Inc.

Roemer, M.I.
1969 The Organization of Medical Care under Social Security. Geneva: International Labor Office.

1976 Cuban Health Services and Resources. Washington: Pan American Health Organization.

1977 Comparative National Policies on Health Care. New York: Marcel Dekker.

Ronaghy, H.A. and S. Solten
1974 Is the Chinese "Barefoot Doctor" Exportable to Rural Iran. The Lancet. June. 29:1331-1333.

Rosenthal, M. M. and J. R. Greiner
1982 The Barefoot Doctors of China: From Political Creation to Professionalization. Human Organization 41(4):330-341.

Scholl, E. A.
1985 An Assessment of Community Health Workers in Nicaragua. Social Science and Medicine 20(3):207-214.

SECOPS/REGION II (Sub-dvision of Popular Education and Communication in Health/Region II).
1984 Summary Tables. Leon: Nicaragua. Mimeo.

Segall, M.
1983 On the Concept of a Socialist Health System: A Question of Marxist Epsitemology. International Journal of Health Services 13(2):221-225.

Siegel, D.
1985 Task Force Investigates Effects of War on Health Care in Nicaragua. LASA Forum. Austin:Latin American Studies Association, 15(4):44-46.

Starr, P.
1982 The Social Transformation of American Medicine. New York: Basic Books.

Teller, C.
1981 The Demography of Malnutrition in Latin America. Intercom 9(8):8-11.

Ugalde, A.
1979 The Role of The Medical Profession in Public Health Policy Making: The Case of Colombia. Social Science and Medicine 13c:109-119.

1981 Ideological Dimensions of Community Participation in Latin American Health Programs. Paper presented at the Seventh International Conference on Social Science and Medicine, Leeuwenhorst Congress Center, Netherlands. June 22-26,1981.

UNICEF
1983 UNICEF Programme: Nicaragua. Managua, Nicaragua. Mimeo.

UNICEF/WHO Joint Committee on Health Policy
1977 Community Involvement in Primary Health Care: A Study of the Process of Community Motivation and Continued Participation. Twenty-First Session. Geneva:WHO.

UNAG,ATC,CIERA (Union Nacional de Agricultores y Ganaderos UNAG, Asociacion de Trabajadores del Campo ATC, and Centro de Investigaciones y Estudios de la Reforma Agraria CIERA)
1982 Produccion y Organizacion en el Agro Nicaraguense. Managua.

USAID (United States Agency for International Development)
1976 Health Sector Assessment for Nicaragua. Managua: USAID Mission to Nicaragua.

Wolf, E.
1956 Aspects of Group Relations in a Complex Society: Mexico. American Anthropologist 58:1065-1078

WHO(World Health Organization)
1973 Organizational Study on Methods of Promoting the Development of Basic Health Services. Annex II to Official Records of the World Health Organization. Geneva: WHO No. 206 p.110.

Walker, T.
1981 Nicaragua: Land of Sandino. Boulder, Colo.: Westview.

1982 Nicaragua in Revolution. Thomas Walker, ed. New York: Praeger.

1984 The Nicaragua-US Friction: The First Four Years (1979-1983), Part I. Mesoamerica 3(4):8-11.

Wallace, A. F. C.
1956 Revitalization Movements. American Anthropologist 58.

Williams, H.
1984 An Uncertain Prognosis: Some Factors May Limit Progress in the Nicaraguan Health Care System. Medical Anthropology Quarterly 15(3):72-73.

WHO/UNICEF (World Health Organization, United Nations Children's Fund)
1978 Primary Health Care. Report of the International Conference on Primary Health Care, Alma-Ata, USSR, September 6-12, 1978, p.6.

INDEX

Adams, Richard, 21
Agrarian reform, 24, 84; Agency (INDRA), 40
Agricultural workers, Association of (ATC), 29
AID. *See* United States Agency for International Development
Armed Services. *See* Military
Association of Agricultural Workers (ATC), 29, 40
Associations. *See* Women; Children; Health Workers; Parents; Peasants; Workers; Youth
Atlantic coast, 27, 43, 88, 89

Barricada, La (Managua), 41
Birthrate, 57
Booth, John, 21, 23
Borge, Tomas, 64, 65
Bossert, Thomas, 21, 99
Breastfeeding, 70, 73, 80, 82. *See also* Maternal child care
Brigadista. *See* Primary care worker
Bureaucracies, governmental: under Somoza, 25; under the Sandinistas, 39, 61

Campaigns, health. *See* Popular health days
Cara al Pueblo, 27
Casualties, 23, 52, 94
Center for Investigations and Studies of the Agrarian Reform (CIERA), 85
Central America, 11, 93
Childbirth, 41. *See also* Midwives
Children, Association of Sandinista Children (ANS), 29; diseases of 70, 74; impact of health programs on, 56, 57, 92, 94
China, health programs in, 61
Chinandega, hospital in, 46; midwifery program in, 56; health reform seminar in (1976), 16–18, 25
Chorotega, village of: before the revolution, 18–20; after the revolution, 59–60
Churches, 19, 60, 88
Civil Defense Committees (CDC), 26, 27
Clinics. *See* Health clinics

Clinic team, 91
Clinical medicine, 95
Communicable diseases, 16, 31, 35; prevention of, 61, 91; measles, 10, 11, 94, 100; diphtheria, pertussis and tetanus, 11, 60. *See also* Polio
Communist takeover, 18
Community organization, 91, 93. *See also* Participation
Comprehensive Plan for Assistance to Health Areas (PIAAS): manual, 90, plan, 87, 90, 92, 95
Confederation of Sandinista Workers (CST), 27, 40
Contras, 52, 94, 100, 101
Control of health services: by community 93; by professionals, 7
Councils. *See* Health Committees (before 1979); Popular Health Councils (after 1979)
Cuba, 61, 96
Culture, popular, 79. *See also* Education, popular
Curanderos. *See* Folkhealers

Deaths, 70, 100; infant mortality, 10, 57, 100
Decoding, 70, 74, 79
Dentistry: dental care, 74, 76; dental encounters, 55
Defense, 101
Dengue, 31
Deprofessionalization, 100
Dialogue, 67
Diarrhea, 11, 26, 57, 70, 82
Diseases, 16, 31, 35, 59; prevention of, 61, 91; measles, 10, 11, 94, 100; diptheria, pertussis and tetanus, 11, 60. *See also* Polio
Division of Communication and Popular Education in Health (DECOPS): and assistance to Honduras, 94; health education policies of, 26, 43, 67, 68, 85, 87; and popular health campaigns, 29, 31, 37, 43; and primary health care, 26, 88, 90, 91, 95; and popular health councils, 27, 39, 43

151

Division of Primary Care, 87, 96
Diptheria, pertussis and tetanus (DPT), 11, 33, 35, 60
Draft, compulsory military, 24
Drunkenness, 79

Earthquake, 12, 23
Eduardo del Rio (pseud: Rius), 85
Education, 24, 25, 59, 65, 89; banking education, 65, 66; Ministry of, 59; popular, 65, 66, 67; political 84, 90; problem-posing education, 65. *See also* Health education; Division of Communication and Popular Education in Health
Education workers, 65, 100
Educators, National Association of Nicaraguan (ANDEN), 29
Elling, Ray, 3, 100
Elsberg, Mary, 89, 97
Epidemiological indicators, 43
Escudero, Jose Carlos, 21
Esteli, 20, 21, 43, 56
Evaluation, 29, 92

Farms, 90, 95
Factories, 95
Fanon, Frantz, 64–67
Federation of Health Workers (FETSALUD), 27, 40
Folkhealers, 10, 21, 41, 42, 62
Folktales, 79
Food: price policies for, 60; production of, 62; supplementary feeding programs, 57
Freire, Paulo, 65–68, 84

Gamer, Robert, 21
Garfield, Richard, 21, 100
Guerrillas, 18
Goiter, 11, 57, 59
Government. *See* Nicaraguan goverment; U.S. government
Greaves, Thomas, 21
Guido, Lea, 43, 95, 96. *See also* Minister of Health

Haug, Marie, 4
Health administration, 41, 42, 92, 96
Health areas, 37
Health assemblies, 89
Health brigades, 89
Health brigadista. *See* Primary care worker
Health care. *See* Primary health care; Hospitals
Health clinics: before the revolution, 15, 16; during the insurrection, 24, 26

Health clinics, subsequent to the revolution: construction, 52, 54; in rural village of El Carmen, 41; medical encounters in, 53; and medical personnel, 37, 39, 40–42; and primary care workers, 67, 87, 89; and referrals, 84, 89, 90–91; services in, 37, 38, 46, 56, 62; as targets of the contras, 94, 100
Health committees, 19, 20
Health conditions: after the revolution, 56–59; class differences of, 70; under Somoza, 10, 11, 21
Health coordinators, 26, 67, 68
Health councils. *See* Popular health councils
Health delivery system, 20, 60, 63, 87, 91. *See also* Primary health care
Health education: implementation, 82, 84, 89, 90, 95, 99; philosophy of, 67, 74, 82, 91; as political education, 79, 84; and primary health care, 62; under Somoza, 17, 20. *See also* Freire, Paulo
Health educators: after the revolution, 26; on the Atlantic coast, 89, 90; organization of, 67, 91, 93; role of, 69, 89, 94; under Somoza, 17
Health facilities, 16, 25, 56, 94, 100. *See also* Health clinics; Hospitals
Health financing: fee for services, 74; financial constraints, 61; under Somoza, 9, 11
Health personnel: evaluation by popular health councils, 39, 41, 42; distribution of, 46; training of, 40, 93; utilization before the revolution, 15. *See also* Health workers; Physicians
Health planning, 25, 27, 29; popular health councils and, 38, 39, 56, 82, 95; under Somoza, 12, 13
Health professionals: dominance by, 4, 42, 84; in other countries, 95; inaccessibility, 61, 74; institutional interests, 61, 87; and primary care workers, 89, 90, 92, 93; as a professional class, 5
Health, principles of health care, 25, 43, 61, 96, 100
Health regions, 27, 37
Health sector: assessment of (1976), 10, 12, 14, 18; competing interests in, 84; popular participation in, 38, 39, 42, 88, 100
Health system, changes within, 2, 95, 99, 100; principles, 25; under Somoza, 18, 20
Health workers, 43, 87, 89, 92, 95, 100. *See also* Primary care workers; Health professionals; Health personnel; Multipliers; Federation of Health Workers

Index 153

Hospitals: damage to, 24, 82; capacity, 49, 50; medical encounters in, 52, 53, 56, 62; new constructions of, 46, 56, 84, 96, 100; rebuilding of, 39, 42, 46; hospital stores, 26; under Somoza, 13, 14, 26, 82; usage since 1979, 49
Honduras: border area with, 56, 94; Ministry of Health of, 94

Insurrection: effects on health care, 23–26; health role of the "los muchachos," 82
International Health Organizations: advisors of, 90; agencies of, 97
Institute of Nutrition for Central America and Panama (INCAP), 10, 21
Insurrection, 23–26, 29, 100
Immunizations, 58, 62, 91, 100

Junta of the Government of National Reconstruction. *See* Nicaraguan government
Jara, Oscar, 84, 85

Korten, David, 6
Knowledge: scientific 68; health, 88, 93

Latrines, 57
Learning, 69. *See also* Education
Literacy, 79. *See also* National Literacy Crusade

Malaria control, 31, 32, 43, 57, 58, 79
Malnutrition, 10, 57
Managua, 10, 21, 23, 43
Marfan, Miguel, 85
Marines, U.S., 23
Matagalpa, 20, 21, 43
Maternal child care, 62, 91, 92; breastfeeding, 70, 73, 80, 82; oral rehydration, 57, 74, 78; mother–child primary care workers, 92, 94; mother mortality, 10; prenatal and postpartum care, 56, 94; role of AMNLAE. *See also* Midwives
Measles, 10, 11, 33, 35, 94, 100
Medical encounters, 44, 53, 56
Medical instruction, office of, 93
Medical profession, 4, 5
Medical professionals, 91, 93, 95 *See also* Physicians
Medical schools, 97
Medical students, 37, 97
Medicines, 26, 62, 91, 93
Midwives, 10, 16, 21, 21n, 56, 90, 92
Military, 5, 79, 100, 101. *See also* militia

Militia, 24, 79
Minister of Health, 42, 43, 95, 96
Ministry of Health (MSP) under Somoza, 9, 10, 13, 14, 16, 18
Ministry of Health (MINSA) under the Sandinistas: and folkhealers, 41, 62; and Honduras, 94; and midwives, 56; policy conflicts within, 5, 6, 26, 29, 31, 38, 42, 43, 87, 90, 93–96; and popular health councils, 29, 40, 63; and popular health days, 31, 37, 38, 90; and the private sector, 46, 59; and regionalization 31; reorganization of, 90, 93. *See also* Division of Communication and Popular Education in Health (DECOPS)
Ministry of Planning, 87
Miskitu, 88
Moravians, 89
Morbidity, 10, 11
Mortality, 10, 57, 70, 100
Multipliers, 32, 67, 69, 89. *See also* Health workers
Municipio (County), 21, 37, 40

National Agricultural Program (INVIERNO), 18
National Guard, 12, 23, 25, 82, 88
National Literacy Crusade, 59, 64, 65, 67, 69, 84, 89
National Peasant League (UNAC), 40
National policies: austerity (1981), 43; emergency plan (1980), 27; health (1976), 16; health (1979), 3, 25, 43; regionalization (1982), 27
National Sanitation Plan (PLANSAR–1977), 15, 16, 18–20
National Unified Health System (SNUS): antecedents, 18; constituencies within, 7, 26, 39; foundation of, 3, 24, 25; policies of, 43; and primary health care workers, 92
Nationalized health system, 4, 5, 100
National University (UNAM), 40
Navarro, Vicente, 4
Neighborhoods, 90, 95
Nicaragua: literacy rate in, 25; map of, 28; medical professionals in, 5; occupation by United States Marines, 23; rural communities in, 60; under Somoza, 23, 24
Nicaraguan government: accountability of, 60, 61, 100; organization of people, 27, 29, 84; regional structure, 31; under Somoza, 18, 20. *See also* National policies

Nicaraguan health system. *See* Health system
Nicaraguan revolution: negotiations within, 7, 99; health in, 20, 25, 43; lessons of, 61, 63; pressures on, 96, 100
Nueva Segovia, 20
Nurses, 25, 42, 92. *See also* Health workers
Nutrition, 57, 62, 91

Occupation health, 92
Oral rehydration, 57, 74, 78
Oral vaccine, 94
Organizations. *See* Popular organizations
Outreach programs, 84. *See also* Primary health care

Panama, 6
Pan American Health Organization, 87
Parents, 70; Association (APF), 29
Parteras. *See* Midwife
Participation: ideological interpretation of, 6; and political legitimation of the state, 6; and professional control, 4, 7, 39, 93; revolutionary priority of, 5; and the state, 6; under Somoza, 14. *See also* Health sector
Patients: clinical care of, 41; referrals of, 52, 84, 88; scheduling of, 46
Patron-clientism, 12, 21n, 60
Peasants, Association of Agricultural Workers (ATC), 29
Pechersky, Graciela, 38
Pertussis, 11, 33, 35
Pharmaceuticals. *See* Medicines
Physicians, 38, 42, 91, 93, 95, 96; attrition among, 96; clinical care by, 37, 41, 42, 46; cultural authority, 68; distribution of, 47; in the insurrection, 5, 25, 26; institutional priorities of, 26; and the MINSA, 100; and deprofessionalization, 100; and relationship to non-physicians, 84, 92, 97; and relationship with the FSLN, 96; training of, 95; under Somoza, 15, 21
Picture code, 69
Polio, 33, 35: assistance to Honduras to combat outbreak of, 37; clinical vaccination for, 37; local vaccination programs for (1982), 60; National vaccination programs for (1979), 26; national vaccination programs for (1981), 31; outbreaks of (1951–1979), 11, 16; popular education about, 74, 77; regional vaccination programs for (1983), 94
Popular approaches to health care: 88, 90, 91, 93, 94, 99, 100
Political economy, 9, 20, 25, 100
Popular health campaigns. *See* Popular health days

Popular health commissions. *See* Popular health councils
Popular health councils (CPS): the Division of Communication and Popular Education in Health and, 90, 95; education and, 69; health delivery and, 40, 63, 91, 92; health planning and, 38, 39, 56, 82, 95; health professionals and, 37–40, 42, 46; the experience of the Atlantic coast of, 89; organization of, 27, 29, 30, 39, 61, 74, 82
Popular heath days (JPS): effects of, 87, 99; the experience on the Atlantic coast of, 89; origins of, 5, 29; organization of, 29, 31, 39, 69, 89; problems during, 37, 38, 40, 42, 60
Popular health documents, 63, 69, 82. *See also* Appendix B, 133
Popular health pamphlets: description of, 70–83; illustrators of, 85; objectives of, 63; uses of, 32, 69. *See also* Appendix A, 103
Popular organizations: folkhealers and, 41, 62; government agencies and, 31, 84; health delivery and, 63, 84, 88, 91; health policy and, 25, 63; the experience on the Atlantic coast of, 89; popular health councils and, 39, 63; the Sandinista party and, 27. *See also* Agricultural workers; Children; Health workers; Parents; Peasants; Workers; Youth
Population, effect of increase on health, 57
Practical Concepts, Inc., 14
Prevention of illness: and popular health care, 88, 91, 92; and popular organizations, 82, 83
Primary care workers: delivery of services by, 32, 38, 89–94; health education by, 69, 74, 89–93; relationship of physicians to, 37, 87, 89–93, 95; selection of, 40, 89–93; supervision of, 92; training of, 31, 39, 40, 42, 67, 88–94; types of, 92; under Somoza, 16, 17, 19, 20, 22, 59. *See also* Health workers
Primary health care: conflict in approaches to, 95; definitions of, 62; differences in experiences on the Pacific and Atlantic coasts regarding, 89; Division of primary care, 6, 90, 93; effect of the contra war on, 91; international recognition of successes in, 87; the popular model of, 88, 90–94, 99, 100; program expansion of, 43. *See also* Comprehensive plan for assistance to health areas (PIAAS)
Professionals. *See* Health professionals
Protestants, 19, 88, 91

Rabies, 26, 57, 58
Rama Indians, 88

Refugees, 93
Rehydration. *See* Oral rehydration
Rius, 85
Rural collaborator. *See* Primary care worker
Rural community health program (PRACS–1973), 15–20, 22
Rural community health services grant (1973), 15
Rural health institutional development grant, 15
Rural mobile health program (PUMAR–1965), 15, 16
Rural population, 93, 101

Salt: iodized, 59; mines, 50; rehydration salts, 57
Sandinista army, 5. *See also* Military
Sandinista Defense Committee (CDS): accountability and, 61; Chorotega's CDS, 59, 60; director of, 37, 60; health delivery and, 26, 67, 92; organization of, 27; popular health days and, 37, 38; primary health care worker selection and, 40
Sandinista Front of National Liberation (FSLN): leadership in, 43, 96; membership in, 40; Ministry of Health and, 61, 62; origins of, 21; physicians and, 96; assemblies of, 40
Sandinista police, 5, 60
Sandinista radio, 82
Sandinista revolution: agrarian reform and, 24; decentralization and, 99; defense of, 24; education and, 25; health and, 24, 26; priorities of, 5, 20
Sandinista sympathizers, 20
Sandinista youth, 29
Sanitation: campaigns, 31; food, 58; inspections, 57, 58; programs, 57, 91, 92; workers, 92. *See also* National Sanitation Plan (1977)
Schools: enrollment in, 25; primary care workers in, 90, 92, 95; students in traditional schools, 65
Segall, Malcolm, 3
Sewage disposal, 11, 62
Social medicine, 82
Social security institute (INSS), 9, 12, 13
Social welfare board (JLAS), 13
Socialism: health system and, 3, 4; national goals and, 5, 7
Somoza dictatorship: economics of, 5, 12, 24; health programs under, 15, 16; health reforms under, 16–18, 20; history of, 12, 23; local appointees of, 19, 59, 60; overthrow of, 21, 23; portrayals of, 70, 74, 79, 82; strategic use of health services by, 18, 19, 88

Soviet Union: health system of, 4; health assistance from, 46
Sumu Indians, 88
Surgical care, 52, 94

Taboada, Eugenio, 100
Teachers. *See* Educational workers
Tellez, Dora Maria, 96. *See also* Minister of health
Tetanus, 11, 33, 35, 100. *See also* DPT
Themes, generative, 69
Training. *See* Primary care workers, training of
Treasury, national, 23
Triage, 46
Tuberculosis, 57, 58

UNICEF: assistance in primary care by, 43, 87; birthing kits provided by, 56; recognition of Nicaragua's health successes by, 6. *See also* International health organizations
United Nations, 23
United States: economic boycott by, 93; occupation of Nicaragua by, 23; undeclared war by, 100
United States Agency for International Development (USAID): health program loans from, 15, 16, 18, 21; health sector assessment by (1976), 10, 14, 18, 21; health reform recommendations by (1976), 16, 18, 20, 25

Vaccination posts, 37, 52
Vaccination programs, 16, 31, 32, 60. *See also* Popular health days
Vaccinations: doses of provided, 33; education for, 63; follow-up to, 37; organization for, 43; number of persons vaccinated, 32, 33. *See also* Popular health days
Vertigal integration, 88
Verticality, 21
Visual code, 70. *See also* Education

Waste disposal, 57
Water: potable water programs under Somoza, 11, 74, 75, 91; potable water programs after the revolution, 57, 62; test samples of, 57
Whooping cough, 11, 33, 35
Wolf, Eric, 21
Women: in leadership, 95; roles, 79, 80. *See also* maternal child care
Women, National Association of Nicaraguan Women, "Luisa Amanda Espinoza" (AMNLAE), 27, 37, 40, 41, 56, 67
Workers, Confederation of Sandinista (CST), 27